AF855068

Volume 1

Some Important Medical Sh*t:
Diverticulosis & Diverticulitis

HOW TO AVOID POOPING INTO A PLASTIC BAG
FOR THE REST OF YOUR LIFE

PROFESSOR JONATHAN M. SACKIER

JOHN F. HUNT, MD

DR. NIGEL D. GUEST

Some Important Medical Sh*t: Diverticulosis & Diverticulitis

First Edition

Copyright © 2025 Reticular Formation, DBA Join the Docs. All rights reserved.

Published by JoinTheDocs

No part of this publication may be reproduced, stored in a retrieval system, or transmitted in any form or by any means—electronic, mechanical, photocopying, recording, or otherwise—without the prior written permission of the copyright holders, except in the case of brief quotations embodied in critical articles or reviews.

Disclaimer

The information contained in this book is provided for educational and entertainment purposes only. No warranties, express or implied, are made regarding the accuracy, completeness, or applicability of the content. The author and publisher are not engaged in rendering legal, financial, medical, or other professional advice. Readers are encouraged to consult qualified professionals before acting on any information or techniques described herein.

By reading this book, you agree that neither the author nor the publisher shall be held liable for any loss, damage, or adverse consequences—direct or indirect—arising from the use or misuse of its content, including errors, omissions, or inaccuracies. You are solely responsible for your own choices, actions, and results.

ISBN: 979-8-9998873-0-6

Cover Design by: Robin Cott

Acknowledgements

We are grateful for the support of our friends and colleagues who read and critiqued our manuscript, and for laughing with us, and not at us. Thanks to Robin Gott for his brilliant doodles and to John Flynn for converting the manuscript from crayon to craftsmanship.

We would never have completed this manuscript without the diligent efforts of Phil Deschamps, who served as publisher, business manager and general good fellow.

Thank you to Nicole Deschamps for her invaluable advice to develop the audiobook.

Individually, John would like to thank Kimmie, Nigel appreciates Christine's support, and Jonathan appreciates his Muse for encouraging and supporting him. All unselfishly allow us to embarrass ourselves.

And finally, we appreciate the medical systems of the UK and US for being generally daft and flatulent.

Contents

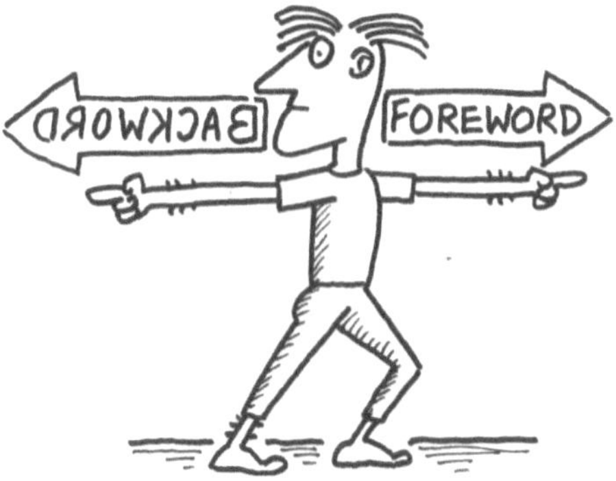

Foreword

The purpose of this book is to take you on a journey from your mouth to your anus: now that's a thought to ponder. Time to get your head out your arse, and your brain into your bowel! Your gut is a long and complex tube, with multiple components ensuring the bowels are beautifully and intelligently suited to the job at hand, extracting goodness from food and providing gainful employment to sanitation engineers.

If it sounds odd to be using words like *beautiful* when referring to bowels, let me explain: as a surgeon I have spent many years studying the human body when healthy and *all* of it is beautiful. I then spent many more years learning about what happens when it all goes wrong, how to recognize and treat beastly diseases. Beauty and the Beast.

This book, and the others to follow, were inspired by a love of medicine that I share with my co-authors and dear friends, Dr. John Hunt and Dr. Nigel Guest. We were due to have a catch-up chat one day when John apologized that he could not join, having just been stricken with a bout of *diverticulitis,* the topic of this volume.

When he recovered, it became apparent that if a bright spark like John had his head up his arse about this disease, maybe others were clueless as well, and the concept for the *Important Sh*t* books was born.

Who is this book series for? Well, if you have a pulse and can read you are our target audience! This specific volume? Adults who have a pulse, can read, have a gut and don't fancy pooping into a plastic bag attached to their side. Motivated? Read on! After all, diverticulosis (the precursor of diverticulitis) affects more than half of people over age 60, is becoming ever more common, and is largely *preventable.* We'd like to help you prevent it.

People aren't always motivated to do things that may help in the long term, but which seem to have no immediate benefit, such as staying fit. Turns out that they are even worse at *avoiding* things that will have long term negative impacts: smoking, being overweight, any of countless risky behaviours. After all, most of us indeed do have our heads up our arses in that regard. But we can extract our heads occasionally, and that's what we are shooting for in this book.

A bit about myself. I am originally from London but educated in Liverpool. I trained in surgery in Britain before heading to America to help introduce laparoscopic surgery to the colonies, so

I was one of the guys to bring "keyhole" and robotic surgery to the masses. When I'm not up to my neck in someone's intestines, I enjoy flying planes, sailing, scuba diving, skiing, hiking, and cooking. I can also swim, but to be honest, I'd rather be in a hot tub.

As above, I am sharing this adventure with Dr. Nigel Guest, a family doctor from Dudley in the British midlands (which accounts for his bizarre accent that only a mother could love). He's also a Liverpool University alum and has spent his career in the National Health Service (NHS), managing everything from general practice to large-scale healthcare innovations. When not healing the sick, Nigel delights in making asinine puns, irritating me, sailing, swimming, and cooking, but rarely at the same time. His life dream is to witness two red London buses cross in the middle of the iconic Tower Bridge. Pathetic really.

Nigel and I produce a podcast that you may have stumbled across, *Join the Docs* (www.jointhedocs.com) which is available on all the usual podcast platforms. In much the same way that this book delivers news-you-can-use with a touch of humour, our podcast does the same. We believe laughter truly is the best medicine (although we are never laughing at our patients or their disease.) But mind you, we might laugh at our colleagues. Actually, we *do* laugh at our colleagues.

And importantly, please also meet Dr. John Hunt, our long-suffering diverticulitis patient and paediatrician, allergologist, pulmonologist and immunologist. A lot of *-ist's* that basically mean he is damn smart. Except about diverticulitis! He is also a diver and sailor, but his time with the American Navy meant he likes bigger boats than Nigel and I. He is also a businessman, investor, inventor and author. His *High Ground* novels (written with the famous Doug Casey) are a cracking good read. Check them out. John believes that medical care should involve a discussion between the doctor and patient, and anyone with an MBA should butt out of other people's butts. John has written this book with me, adding his personal experiences and very particular world view.

We thought that three doctors who share a similar sense of humour and a desire to live life with passion, to learn, to discuss and to laugh, might be able to raise awareness about important shit, and go some way to make our profession redundant. Let's face it, we are all patients sooner or later, as John has so ably demonstrated.

Some people believe we doctors think we know it all. The reality is that we don't, and we don't even think we do. To quote the ancients, Nosce te ipsum – "know thyself." We know what we know and always yearn to know more. Some of what we know we can impart to you. You can combine this information with what you know about yourself, and that's a winning combo. So join us on this journey!"

In each volume we shall address a specific topic, cover all the important shit we think will interest you, provide ideas on how to avoid conditions if possible, and what to do if avoidance fails—including questions to ask your care provider, and important resources. Each book will have one of us as primary author with medical expertise contributed from the other two. Or in Nigel's case, contributions of daft jokes. Additionally, we are including doodles by our wonderful friend, Robin Gott. The good artist sees the world through a different lens. We expect his cartoons will make you smile.

We shall be donating a percentage of proceeds from these books and associated products to relevant medical charities.

What we will *not* be doing is scaring you with medical jargon or boring you with dry facts. No, we will scare you with regular words and bore you with wet facts. We want to educate you in a way that's engaging and easy to understand. Plus, we'll share some real-life stories from our own practices to illustrate key points. We will not be hawking branded vitamins or any other form of snake oil, just medical facts that three experienced doctors from different specialties know at the time of writing. Of course, medical knowledge changes with time and any errors that arise can be corrected in future editions. In this regard, we were told that within five years of graduating from medical school, 50% of what we had been taught will be proven to be wrong; the challenge is knowing which 50%! And given how long it is since we were at university, pretty much everything we learned there is wrong. Fortunately, we kept learning the newest and most up-to-date stuff during our careers.

In this book, we shall travel the bowel in all its winding glory... that's windy (as in twisty, not windy as in farting, although everyone farts, even royalty, but it presumably has a rather more polite sound and delicate aroma). We shall then dig into the colon, metaphorically of course, as I am sure you wouldn't want to be elbow deep in real shit! We will then explain what happens that leads to diverticulitis. Given our very own Dr. Hunt is a patient, we shall have the perspective of someone who has suffered from the symptoms, and if I have my way, will experience some of the surgical wizardry my branch of medicine has to offer.

In future books I cannot guarantee that one of us will conveniently suffer from the relevant ailment, but Nigel has gamely offered to try and get pregnant so he can talk us through that experience!

In full disclosure, I am both British and American, spent half my life in the USA and have deep affection for the country and its people, but George Bernard Shaw said the US and Britain were two nations divided by a common language, so we must choose a spelling and grammatical style and stick to it. Nigel is also English, is bigger than John and cannot understand American English, so we are going with the British version. To our American readers, we apologize for seemingly endless bizarre spellings.

If you want to write to us with comments, suggestions for other topics you want us to cover or to say nice things, please send an email or direct message to John, Nigel or myself (see below). And if you want to say something nasty, we would rather you did not, but if you must, please only heckle us in Latin or Greek – after all, we want to put our education to work.

We also want to thank Phil Deschamps for his leadership in keeping John, Nigel and yours truly in check, and every doctor back to Hippocrates and Galen for their contributions to keeping us all alive.

Finally, please bear in mind that a book can never replace a face-to-face interaction with a medical professional. These tomes are intended to educate and entertain and do not imply that you, dear reader, and the authors of this volume have forged a doctor-patient relationship. Guess how much we had to pay our lawyers to come up with that disclaimer.

Professor Jonathan M Sackier

London, England, August 2025

info@jointhedocs.com

Instagram, Tiktok, Facebook, YouTube: @jointhedocs

1

Colon Quest

The Final Digestination

Introduction

Let's start with a question that may never have crossed your mind while munching on a cheeseburger; *"how did that yummy meal keep me going and turn itself into poop?"* The answer lies in the glorious magic of your digestive tract, a biological dis-assembly line whose elegant complexity we shall endeavour to explain. After all, if you can appreciate how muesli becomes muscle, maybe it will change how, and what, you eat.

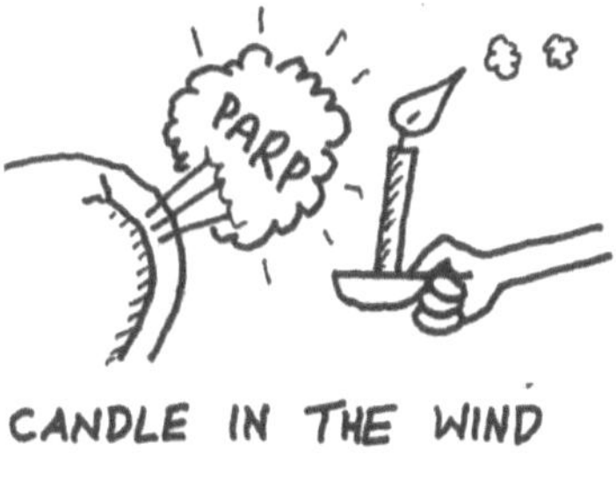

CANDLE IN THE WIND

Anatomy professors may tell you that the human hand and its opposable thumb is the most brilliant bit of evolutionary invention. Forgive the image, but the human hand doesn't hold a candle to the brilliance of lower human bowels, even illuminated by a candle. Not that we are suggesting you hold a flame to your nether regions.

Try to imagine holding in your outstretched hand, palm down, a mixture of solids, liquids and gases. Now, through an act of will alone, try to release only the gas. It would be an amazing feat. But where the hand fails, the rectum and its mate, the anus, routinely succeeds in an act celebrated by young men the world over, especially after a few beers. The rectum is clearly superior to the long-admired hand, but less often adorned by varnish or jewelry.

For just a moment, imagine the famed French flatulist Joseph Pujol (yes, his name is pronounced Poo-hole) who went by the stage name Le Pétomane, French for "farting maniac" because literally, his act was to fart at will. Had he not possessed a talented lower bowel, the performance assuredly would not have been well-attended.

To navigate a maze, one is often advised to place your left hand on one wall and keep following around to the centre, as it is one continuous surface. When speaking of the gut, the phrase "mouth-to-anus" comes to mind, and perhaps it is disquieting to realize that the gut is one continuous surface. So, the next time you kiss someone, or pop something in your pie-hole, you are close to touching your tailpipe. If you kiss someone's arse, you could double the length of that maze. And kissing each other's arse would make a loop.

But what are the various bits and pieces from mouth to anus, and what do they do? Understanding that will help everything fall into place. (Pooping, falling into place. Haha! Only the puerile mind would go straight to the toilet with that line, but we doctors have nothing if not puerile minds.) So, Anatomy 101, or as Olivia Newton-John might have said, let's get intestinal!

Anatomy & physiology: The parts of your gut and what they do

When aromatic food appeals, the gut serves to take such delightful delicacies and turns them into energy and waste whose aroma most decidedly does not appeal. In the 007 film, *Diamonds are Forever*, Bond has hidden jewels in a deceased villain's gastrointestinal tract and tells his colleague the decision was "alimentary." The gut is about 30 feet (9 metres) long to accomplish all the tasks it has before it. Just another three men talking about length, but here it's not compensating for anything. The alimentary tract consists of the following parts and merit an alliterative aperitif – check out Figures 1 and 2 as you read along:

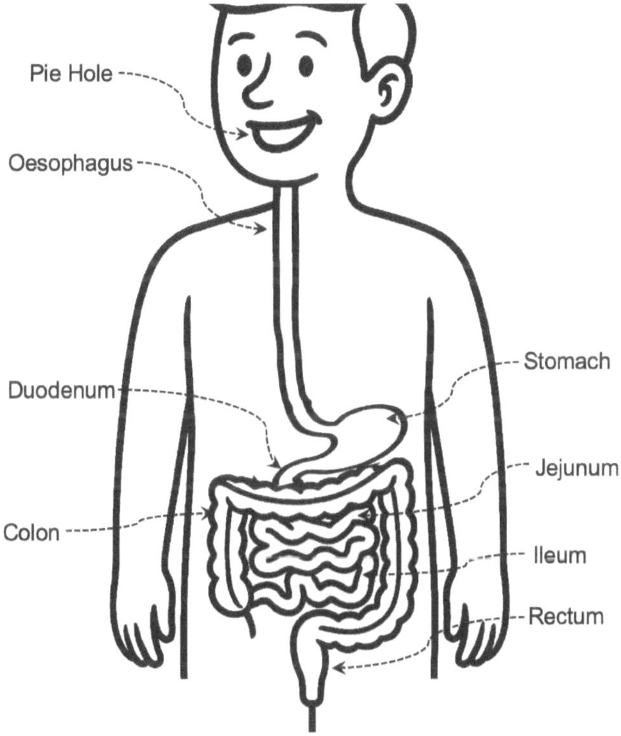

Figure 1. Normal gut anatomy

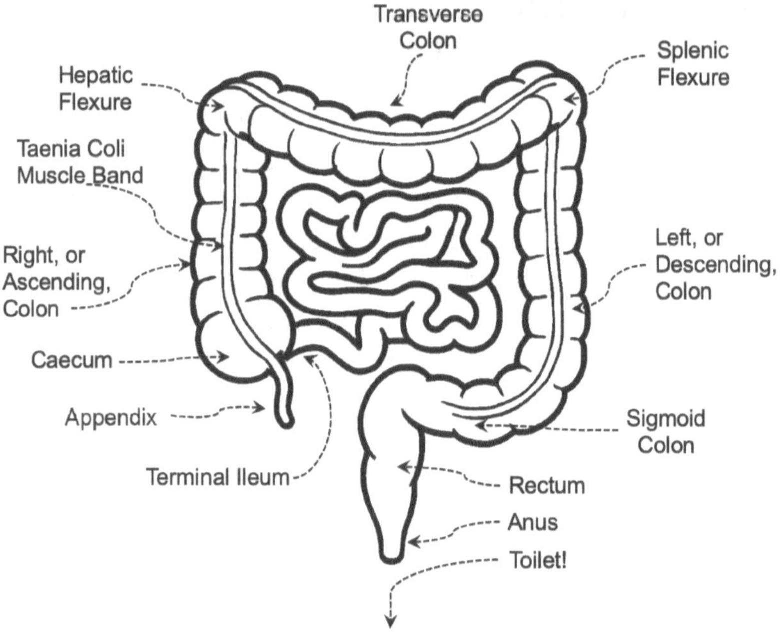

Figure 2. Looking closer at the abdominal gut anatomy

- In the mouth, saliva lubricates and breaks down delicacies with the aid of *mastication* (fancy word for chewing), to be distinguished from masturbation which should not be done in a restaurant.
- Once swallowed, overcome oatmeal enters the oesophagus (gullet) as the first waves of peristalsis (coordinated contraction) move the food into the....
- Stomach, a muscular bag where subdued sausage is assailed by enough acid to consume the most belligerent of James Bond's foes and further pummeled by peristalsis and powerful pepsin, a digestive enzyme. Then ...
- The *duodenum* further deploys destructive force delivered from the *pancreas* with an enzyme called *amylase* to conquer carbohydrates, another called *lipase* to liberate fat, and another named *trypsin* to pulverize protein. The liver kicks in

bile which does all sorts of clever things (tune in to future volumes) including freeing fats from food. In case you are interested, the duodenum gets its name from Latin (I know, big surprise) and means "twelve finger breadths" because that is about how long it is. Fascinating, right?

- Next up – or rather down from the duodenum is the *jejunum,* also Latin and meaning "empty" because when Greek doctors first dissected dead people they found this part of the intestine did not contain any food or fluid. It is known for absorbing iron, but mostly just moves things along to the next part of the bowel. It also gave rise to the word *jejune* meaning simple or childish. A term often ascribed by us to Nigel.
- And now, partially digested food enters the *ileum,* (the Latin here is boring, just meaning "intestines") a part of the small bowel whose main role is to absorb all the goodies the prior parts of the gut prepared to be absorbed.
- In the bottom right part of the belly, the ileum plugs into the first part of the colon, the caecum: a capacious pouch from which the vermiform appendix dangles (the words mean "attached worm" because the appendix looks similar to a worm). The colon's main purpose is to extract water from poop and move it with peristalsis towards the left side. It is long, around one meter or 3 feet. The entire gut lining makes (and oozes out) mucus, the medical word for snot, a protein and carbohydrate-rich substance that lubricates the passage of poop that becomes more important the further down the bowel we travel. Inside the gut are gazillions (my son assures me that is a real number) of bacteria, known as the microbiome, a colony of critters

> Everyone's microbiome is different, which is one of the many reasons why each person should be treated as an individual as opposed to a statistic, both medically, and in all other settings.

whose role in health and disease is becoming better understood.

- The right-side of the colon ascends towards the rib cage and is very creatively called the right colon or ascending colon. Clever stuff, this medical nomenclature. At the liver it takes a sharp turn to your left and traverses the belly – and you will be astounded to know we called it.... the transverse colon! This transverse colon is high up in the belly, and some is even under the ribcage in the front. It then takes a turn south on the left side of the belly and descends to become, yes, you guessed it, the descending or left colon. Because it is not too keen on leaving just yet, it does a few turns this way and that to look like a letter "S" and we thus have named that next part of it the sigmoid colon.

- Once the stool has navigated those sigmoid "S" turns, it enters the rectum, which is Latin for "straight gut" although the rectum isn't that straight (we use straight as a geometric term here, not a sexual one). The rectum serves to remove that last bit of water and store poop until it is convenient to send stool southward to re-emerge in the world at large. To do this, the rectum has nerves that send messages to the brain suggesting that it would be wise to find a toilet soon. Additionally, when one eats, the gastrocolic reflex sends a message from stomach to the lower bowel basically saying "Oy! You down there, make some room, more poop coming your way!"

> The right side of the colon is where politicians from the right side of the political spectrum keep their heads. The left side of the colon is where politicians from the left side of the spectrum keep theirs. The moderates twaddle along between the two in the transverse colon while having committee meetings.

- The rectum relies heavily on the anal canal and anal sphincter, a short, complex muscular tube that controls the emission of poop, and provides the musicality of farts – more of that later.

With the above information you can see why those doctors who are Beatles fans might think of the bowel as a long and winding road that leads to your door. Or in this case, your anus.

Role of the colon in digestion and health

As noted, the entire bowel exists to digest food with the colon dedicated to desiccating waste and storing it before discharge: one way traffic if you like. Although not always one way, for instance:

1. If prepared correctly, many medications can be delivered rectally, including acetaminophen (Tyleonol in the USA or paracetamol in Britain) and some drugs that stop vomiting. In cases where intravenous administration of fluids is delayed or impossible, medical staff can insert fluids into the colon to rehydrate patients. On July 2nd, 1881, President James Garfield was shot by a lawyer who was unhappy with him. The assault did not kill him immediately and so to treat him, fluids were pumped into his rectum. Alexander Graham Bell—who we hold responsible for irritating people speaking loudly on their phones—tried to find the bullet with a device he developed, but to no avail. Garfield died several weeks later.

2. There is a nasty condition called *pseudomembranous colitis* – any disease with a name that long is bound to be unpleasant; it can lead to the colon turning into a material akin to bleeding wet tissue paper, which is bloody awful and if not treated, tends to be fatal. One way to treat this – and I am not making this up – is a faecal transplant, whereby a healthy donor contributes poop that is dried, treated and either consumed by

the patient or introduced during a colonoscopy. One might say, "Eat shit and don't die!"

3. The term colorectal foreign bodies is not a derisory phrase for immigrants with poor toilet habits, but rather the insertion of various things where the sun don't shine. Originally thought by doctors to be a way to deal with an itchy bottom (we call it pruritus ani because we are too embarrassed to say "itchy bottom" and can charge more for the Latin), this is now generally found in the setting of a search for sexual gratification. For those interested in the range of artificial objects that manage to find their way ("accidently") into the rectum, check out our Further Reading for examples, including a paper written by yours truly documenting 42 cases. Physicians who encounter such an occurrence must always ascertain if the insertion was a function of two - or more - consenting adults or a case of assault or abuse.

> Interestingly, in America, the term to have an accident is used to describe when stuff comes out of the rectum unintentionally.

4. Anal sex of course – no more discussion necessary.

We are what we eat, and so is our stool!

From farm to table, and from table to your arse. The body needs various substances to run, repair and replenish as well as to fight decay and disease. Just as each component of our food impacts how the body works – or doesn't – it also affects the stool, and the stool can affect the body.

For instance, water is required to keep blood at the right consistency, the kidneys working properly, all our cells the right size and shape, and to assure that electrolytes (salts) are maintained at the right concentration to keep the body functioning. We have seen that the colon removes water from waste. If too little water is

> Drink lots of water.

consumed, every system will falter, and stool will be dry and hard causing extra work for the colon, with bad consequences such as painful splits in anal skin, possible abscesses, and ... diverticulosis. If stool contains nasty cancer-causing substances and it sticks around for too long, the chance of developing cancer goes up. You will see throughout this book that we will repeatedly recommend drinking lots of water repeatedly. And we will repeat that recommendation repeatedly.

In the same vein – or colon – fibre is critically important to keep things moving. Fibre stays in the gut because it is not absorbed, serving to maintain stool volume and to hurry digested food through the bowels. One can consume it by eating lots of fresh fruit and vegetables or, more expensively, as a medication. More information on this will follow.

2

Colonic Cul-de-Sacs

Diverticulosis & Diverticulitis

Introduction

So, given the scene we have set in Chapter 1, your bowels silently (other than the odd squeak or toot) go about their daily business, not bothering you except when they need you to find a porcelain throne to "do your business." Until one day they announce their presence by causing discomfort that may turn out to be your introduction to the world of diverticulosis. This refers to the condition where little blind pouches develop in the colon, each of which is called a diverticulum while many are called diverticula. If you want to imagine what this looks like, take an inflated balloon and squeeze it in your hands; you will see little balloon pouches popping out between your fingers – diverticula. Come to think of it, if one doesn't tie the end of an inflated balloon and let it go, it endeavours to resemble the colon in another way! Check out Figure 3 as you work your way through this chapter.

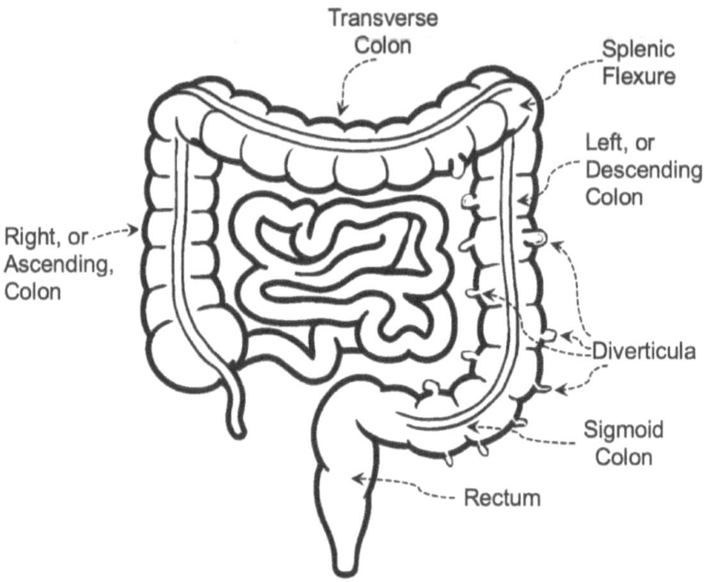

Figure 3. Diveriticula on descending and sigmoid colon

Referring to Anatomy 101 in the prior chapter, the colon travels from caecum to rectum, from the right side to the left side. To push food on its journey, most of the gut is lined by two layers of muscle, one where the fibres run the length of the bowels, another that is wrapped around them in rings. But on reaching the caecum (the beginning of the large intestine), the long fibres split into three bands called *taenia coli* rather than being a continuous layer. It is in these areas (where there is only a circular muscle layer) that blood vessels enter the colon (for the purposes of nourishing the bowel and absorbing water into the bloodstream). These areas tend to be weak spots. It is here that pouches can develop from pressure being too great inside the colon. The proximity of diverticula to arteries will take on greater significance later in our tale. Or tail.

Diverticula are the potholes on your digestive highway, forming when the inner layer of your intestine pushes through weak spots in the muscle wall when slow moving, heavy poop passes through. Rather like slow, heavy trucks damaging the tarmac as they trundle through. Diverticula can occur elsewhere in the gut, either as something one is born with or that develop later in life, but this book is staying firmly in the sewer (or the sections of the gut closest to the sewer). While colonic diverticula can occur from the caecum all the way around to the left side, these sac-like protrusions most commonly pop up in the sigmoid colon, the part of the large intestine closest to your rectum. Sorry to do this, but a little bit more anatomy; once the sigmoid plugs into the rectum, the three long muscle layers join again creating a thick muscular region in the rectum capable of delivering the expulsive force needed to poop. Additionally, the rectum dives under a nice tight tissue blanket called the *peritoneum*. This is why diverticula cannot form in this part of the bowel, but instead tend to occur one section earlier, in the sigmoid colon.

Most people don't even know they have diverticula. You might be sitting there reading this fine and informative book, blissfully unaware that your colon's got a few extra pockets. Think about it: unless you have something in your jacket pocket, you may be blissfully unaware it is there.

Developing diverticulosis

Diverticula formation is a function of diet and lifestyle. Low-fibre diets, common in Western cuisine, are a big part of the problem. Fibre's job is to keep poop bulked up to help things move smoothly. Without fibre, stool is smaller, harder and your colon must push more, thereby, increasing pressure inside the bowel which leads to these diverticular pouches forming. And as noted at the end of Chapter 1, wet poop is good, dry poop not so much. So, while you might love your steak and potatoes, your colon might be dreaming of beans and whole grains. These little pouches are usually harmless, unless they decide to throw a tantrum, which is what we'll explore next.

Imagine a row of nice, neat houses, a peaceful neighbourhood with everyone minding their own business. And then someone decides to build a glassed-in sunroom extension sticking out into their garden, and folks on the street are concerned how this might change things. Diverticulosis is like that, when first one, then another house pops out an extension. The strange appearance may generate some odd looks from people driving through town, but no harm, no foul.

Most people live with diverticulosis without ever knowing. It's the silent shy type, lurking in the shadows of your digestive tract, occasionally found as part of a medical checkup such as in a routine colonoscopy. However, diverticulosis can be the cause of vague or intermittent cramping belly pain (most often in the left lower part of the belly) and some bloating. Diverticulosis can lead to infrequent bowel movements, a sense of incomplete emptying, and excretion of numerous small chunks of stool (although these are also often due to the diet that causes diverticulosis in the first place, rather than the diverticulosis itself).

How common is diverticulosis?

Historically, diverticulosis wasn't even on the radar until the 20th century. In the early 1900s, people ate high-fibre diets, and diverticulosis and its sequel, diverticulitis, was virtually unheard of. Fast forward to the late 20th and 21st centuries and blammo, we've got a surge in cases. Blame it on our couch potato habits, sedentary lifestyles and longer lifespans, but let's not fail to indict our modern love affair with processed foods.

The prevalence of diverticulitis has increased significantly over the years, especially in younger people. A study from the Rochester Epidemiology Project found that the incidence of diverticulitis nearly doubled from 1980 to 2007. As one of us is a surgeon (JMS) who has practiced on both sides of the Atlantic, I have

> The increased use of CT scans has also contributed to this rise in diagnosis of both asymptomatic diverticulosis and symptomatic diverticulitis, which may not have been noticed before CTs.

welcomed visiting surgeons from African nations (where a high-fibre diet is the norm) who had never seen a case in their country.

Diverticulosis and diverticulitis certainly do not respect status or wealth; From what we read in the terrifically trustworthy on-line media, Pope Francis, wrestler Brock Lesnar, and many other celebrities have suffered with the condition. Hardly surprising given how common it is.

Diverticulitis

Now imagine those glass sunrooms heating up, attracting the owners' drunk and rowdy friends who make a lot of noise and maybe break a pane of glass or two. That's diverticulitis: those quiet little pouches transform into inflamed or infected bags. Basically, what happens is the pouch openings gets blocked by some hard poop and the contained mucus acts as a meal for some trapped crappy bacteria.

> The Americans use the term *pooped* as synonymous with *exhausted*. Those silly Americans!

The affected diverticulum turns into a bucket of pus that, like infection elsewhere in the body, make one feel wretched with fever, nausea and vomiting and a general sense of being ill.

Understanding the difference between these two conditions is crucial. Diverticulosis is often quiet, a symptomless (asymptomatic) colonic companion, whereas diverticulitis is the loud alarm bell, signaling something's gone seriously awry. With diverticulitis, you're more likely to find yourself in the company of one or more doctors – and you will not be having fun. They will be advising you about re-evaluating your diet and life choices, or in worst case scenarios, introducing you to their surgical colleagues (someone like me)! While diverticulosis can be managed with lifestyle adjustments, diverticulitis sometimes requires hospitalization, medications or surgery. One is a passive condition; the other is a call to action that requires more urgent medical intervention.

What causes diverticulosis and diverticulitis?

Genetics: "You look just like your dad!" Or "that musical ability must be genetic!" But you could be inheriting from your family something that you would rather have them leave out of their wills. Genetics play a big role in the development of diverticulosis. Studies suggest that certain inherited genes are the ticket to this intestinal club. So, next time someone compliments your family resemblance, just smile and reply, "Yep, you should see our colons!"

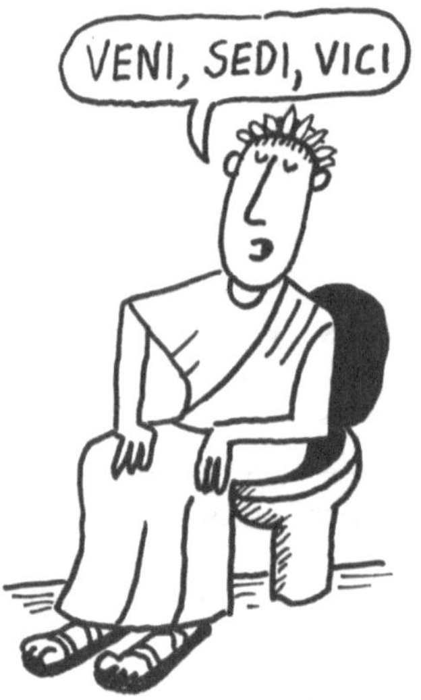

Certain genetic diseases that impact how tissues in the body behave may raise the chances of developing diverticulosis. For instance, *Ehlers-Danlos Syndrome, Polycystic Kidney Disease* and *Marfan's Syndrome* negatively impact the connective tissues (structural support systems that hold organs and tissues together) and therefore cause all manner of mischief. For instance, Ehlers-Danlos causes very flexible joints and Marfan's patients have a tall appearance with other characteristics such as a high-arched palate and a tendency to develop aneurysms. Some famous people had the latter condition including Charles De Gaulle, actor Peter Mayhew (Chewbacca in *Star Wars*) and possibly Julius Caesar and Abraham Lincoln. History does not tell us about Caesar's toilet habits, but maybe they misheard "I came, I saw, I conquered" and Caesar really said, "I came, I sat, I conquered." Who knows. History is mostly made-up shit anyway.

While genetics might hand you a ticket to the diverticulosis show, family history writes the program notes. If you have first-degree relatives (parents or siblings) with the condition, you might find yourself in a similar boat, courtesy of your family tree. Doctors ask you about family medical history for good reason. It gives you a heads-up about what might be lurking around your colon's corner. Additionally, while *nature* plays some role, *nurture* is important: nurture relates to *how* one lives. We will get into that below.

Age: Age is a risk factor for diverticulosis, as your colon wall gets a bit weaker each time you circle the sun and unlike a fine wine, your colon doesn't get better with age. Diverticulosis prevalence skyrockets with age, like the number of candles on your birthday cake. It's estimated that up to half of the population over 65 has diverticulosis, making it a popular club that nobody really wants to join. This results from waning elasticity of colon muscle, making it more susceptible to forming pesky pouches. As we will see below, being active helps limit development of diverticulosis. But aging leads to less physical activity.

Diet: Modern diets, filled with processed delights and red meat, cause the traffic jam referenced above. Imagine your colon being a bit like a pressure cooker. A low-fibre diet is akin to sealing the lid without letting off steam. Over time, pressure builds up until something gives way. Although we have described the intestines as a thing of beauty, the weakness between the bands of muscle is an accident waiting to happen. The pressure encourages diverticula to form, popping out from the wall like kernels of corn expanding with heat. But when these puppies pop, it does not preface a fun night watching a movie. Eating too much red meat and not enough fruits or veggies might not seem like a big deal, but your colon disagrees. It prefers a diet rich in fibre. Without it, the pressure required to push faeces out your bottom increases and the hard pellets of poop can block the entrance to the blind alleys that are your diverticula. That's trouble.

Remember that the colon produces mucus to lubricate the passage of faeces on your southbound carriageway, to the tune of about 400 ml per day. That's about 1 pint, and not the type of warm, strong pint that Brits enjoy in a pub. The colon contains about twenty trillion bacteria. For context, as of December 9th, 2024, the United States government debt was $36.17 trillion – and we know *that* is a big number! To those bacteria, mucus is as appealing as a double cheeseburger with fries and a shake, and they gladly munch down on it. Under normal circumstances, that's just a natural part of the bacterial restaurant inside your bowels. But when a gob of mucus and a bunch of bugs get pushed into and stuck inside a blocked diverticula pouch, things get ugly. Fast. As the bacteria chow down on the sticky goop, gases are released, bugs die, and the deterioration leads to pus forming. Incidentally, for "goop" I am *not* referring to the line of products launched by Gwyneth Paltrow. I am using the word first referenced from *Dialect Notes* in the Oxford English Dictionary in 1914.

One should aim for at least 28 grams of fibre a day. Or maybe 29. Whole grains, fruits and vegetables are the way to go. So, when planning your next food shopping trip, incorporate some high-fibre cereals and raspberries instead of that extra-large bag of chips. Your colon will thank you.

> 28, 29 grams, who cares? No one. The point is to eat more fibre.

Fluid: Another trigger of diverticulitis is consuming insufficient fluids. We will repeat this in the book, a lot: Drinking lots of water keeps stool softer, which then requires less pressure to move down the line, which helps keep diverticulosis from becoming diverticulitis.

Exercise: Spending too much time on the couch is also a risk factor. Exercise stimulates bowel motions thereby ensuring digested food spends less time in your insides and more in the toilet. When you to go to the gym or for a long walk, think of that exercise as contributing to the fitness of your colon as well as your well-toned butt. While your couch might look inviting, your colon's future might depend on a brisk walk or a dance session in your living room. No need to run marathons; just keep your body and your colon in motion.

> In fact, let's repeat this right now. If you have diverticulosis, drink lots more water than the average person!

Stress: This is not good for us in any way, other than being great at inducing *onychophagia*, the fancy word for nail biting. Stress certainly isn't kind to your gut. The *autonomic* part of the human nervous system manages stuff that you don't normally have to think about – breathing, heartbeats and where blood flows to. When we are stressed, the body is focused on *fight or flight*, diverts blood away from the gut and slows the processes detailed in Chapter 1. When we are relaxed, the nervous system goes into a *rest and digest* mode that allows the intestines, colon included, to do their stuff. Stress therefore has the same negative effects as eating less fibre, drinking less water and holding onto one's poop.

> Mind you, for some people a stressful situation can lead to explosive diarrhoea which has some parallels in the animal kingdom. For instance, many creatures, from caterpillars to hippos fling poop when cornered, others, including birds and sloths just lose it if under attack and of course, opossums literally play dead and empty every orifice.

Medications: Certain medications, such as steroids and non-steroidal anti-inflammatory drugs like ibuprofen, can cause trouble for diverticulitis. Although generally well tolerated, ibuprofen can worsen bleeding in acute episodes by interfering with blood clotting. See Appendix III for medications that are important to know about in diverticulosis.

Smoking and Alcohol: This devilish duo of bad habits also contributes to the risk of developing diverticulitis. Smoking promotes inflammation and decreases blood flow. Increased inflammation may make your colon more susceptible to diverticulitis. We will discuss inflammation more in the next chapter. And alcohol? It's not much better. Consuming it in excess can lead to increased risk. So, if you needed another reason to quit smoking or to cut back on the beer, wine or martinis, consider your colon's well-being.

You cannot choose your genetic make-up, but you can avoid these risk factors and doing so could significantly lower your chances of having to deal with diverticulitis.

Pooping: You have learned that increased pressure inside the bowel caused by hard, smaller stool predisposes to the formation of diverticula. If you made a good decision about who your parents were, and follow the above guidance, you are doing much of what you can to reduce the incidence of diverticulosis. However, there is one simple and important trick everyone should follow.

As mentioned above, our body is equipped with an awfully clever control system called the gastrocolic reflex that tells us it is time for a BM. Within 30 minutes of a high fibre breakfast, a glass of water and a coffee, many people know they'll need some toilet action. The worst thing you can do is suppress that urge, jump in your car and head off to work. All that time the faeces is sitting in your rectum getting harder, drier and trickier to expel. So, if you want to be flushed with success,

> And having given your BM the once-over, close the lid before sending the contents on their way – every time one flushes with an open lid, hordes of evil little bacteria are leaping out the loo and onto your clothes, phone … and toothbrush if it is nearby.

listen to your bowels! And before flushing, have a quick look to see what your poop looks like – any blood, mucus or heaven-forbid, writhing worms, or floating stool merit a trip to the doctor.

So, there you have it: the factors that increase your risk of diverticulosis, from genetics to lifestyle choices. Knowledge is power.

Ignoring diverticulosis symptoms can lead to diverticulitis. And that can lead to a series of unfortunate events. We shall explore these and the symptoms they cause in the next chapter.

3

Fifty Shades of Pain

Diverticulitis

Introduction

As we learned earlier, over half of senior citizens live with diverticulosis. For many, they may never know there are belligerent bowel bags lurking in the dark recesses of their colon. But sometimes things take a nasty turn.

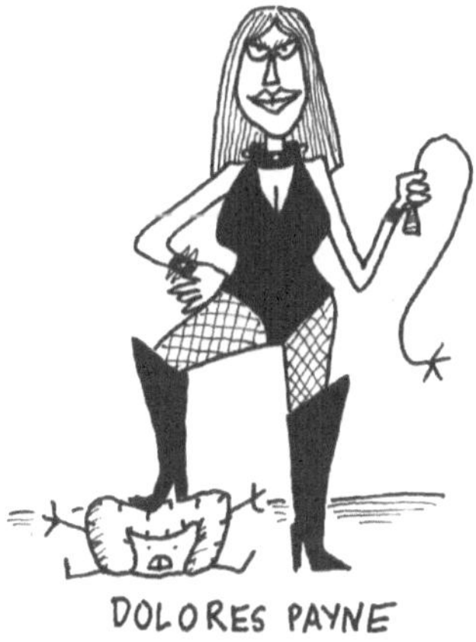

Any time you see the suffix "-itis" think "inflammation," and think in Latin. Specifically, *Calor, Dolor, Rubor, Tumor and functio laesa*. Back in the day in England, a comprehension of Latin was expected of medical school applicants, and although I hated the two years I took, it did come in handy. My teacher was so boring as he took us through declensions, *amo, amas,*

amat and so on that he put himself to sleep. However, it was grand learning to swear in Latin *Te futueo et caballum tuum* for instance – "screw you and the horse you rode in on!" Or *Es mundus excrementi* – "you are a pile of shit!" You see, it gave me *aha* moments; I now knew what excrement meant! And likewise for inflammation, those five items above: *calor* is hot, *dolor* is pain, *rubor* is red, *tumor* is swelling and *functio laesa* is loss of function.

Think about hurting your hand, maybe a burn or nasty cut: it is hot, painful, red, swollen and you cannot use it normally. Same thing if it is an inflamed diverticulum. Hot, red, painful gut swellings impairing how your bowels function.

> And now you know what *inflammation* really means. Rubor, Calor, Dolor and Tumor and some dysfunction. Red, Hot, Painful, Swollen and not working right.

As a diverticulum becomes inflamed, it induces a general sense of being unwell. The presence of infecting bacteria triggers the body to fight back with systemic inflammation (systemic means throughout your whole body, not just your gut). The bacteria can even enter the bloodstream. With a bad episode of diverticulitis, one may experience shivering followed by fever, perspiring, and possibly nausea, vomiting, headache and throbbing abdominal pain. These symptoms will likely be enough that you want to seek medical/professional help. Often everything will settle down on its own but may merit interventions that we will address in Chapters 9 and 10. Such a flare-up may never occur again or may recur often and follow the same or different course. While an experienced patient may recognize the symptoms as their diverticulitis "playing up," it should never be taken for granted as circumstances may take a different turn.

About fevers: When you have an infection, the brain resets your body's thermostat to a higher temperature. The result is that you suddenly feel cold and cover yourself with blankets. The brain's thermostat calls for more heat and so you start shivering. Taking acetaminophen (paracetamol/Tylenol) or ibuprofen will set your temperature on your thermostat back to normal, and this makes you feel hot. You then toss off the blankets and sweat to cool yourself back to normal temperature (called "breaking a fever"). If you want to be more comfortable, don't wait until your temperature is high again to take the next dose of these medications. Instead, take the meds when you *start* feeling cold or start shivering, because you know the fever is coming next.

It is important to note that not everyone will experience the classic symptoms. Many things can influence how diverticulitis shows up. For instance, medications that suppress inflammation –such as steroids taken for rheumatoid arthritis or other conditions—can change how patients experience symptoms. Diverticulitis is a disease more common as we age, and with increased age comes a lower response to infection, and so the fever one usually associates with diverticulitis may not occur.

From another perspective, think how some people react differently to a roller coaster; one is screaming with excitement, the other, holding onto their hat. Gender also plays a role; women might experience bloating and abdominal discomfort that can mimic other conditions, like menstrual cramps, making it tricky to pinpoint the cause. More confusion arises because hormonal fluctuations might impact symptoms. Men often report more straightforward abdominal pain. As your authors are three men, we can state with some certainty that we chaps are rather less stoic than women, who are, regarding pain, the stronger sex for sure. Then there's individual tolerance levels: what might feel like a minor inconvenience to one person could be a full-blown disabling agony for another. Every person's response is as unique as their fingerprints; this individuality in symptom presentation reminds us that our bodies are as unique as our personalities, demanding a personalized approach to management.

Abscess

If the infection does not settle down, pus can build up and form an *abscess,* a swollen area of tissue filled with a pocket of pus. This may present with extreme abdominal pain, a high fever and a sense of being profoundly unwell; basically, worsening symptoms from above. An abscess can also resolve with treatment but may lead to further problems. For instance, it can *perforate* or burst into the general abdominal cavity and lead to *peritonitis,* (as above, "-itis" that is inside the abdominal peritoneal cavity). Given the diverticulum is an outpouching from inside the colon, the pus leaking into the belly compartment can be followed by faeces doing the same. When faeces leak into one's peritoneum and causes peritonitis, it's a life-threatening medical emergency requiring immediate treatment.

Fistula

Sometimes the abscess might stick to the belly wall or another internal organ and subsequently burst through from the gut into some other space, forming a *fistula*. A fistula is an abnormal connection: a tube going from inside the colon to pretty much anywhere else—such as small intestine, bladder or skin—that shouldn't be connected to the colon by a spare tube. A fistula tends to transmit poop in the process to places where it isn't supposed to go. Fortunately, this is not common, but you need to know about it. If the attachment is to the abdominal wall, faeces might start leaking out on to the skin, if into the bladder, one might see "fizzy" urine as air gets into the bladder, *pneumaturia,* and infection in the urine that can spread into the kidneys and cause major illness; Figure 4 illustrates what this looks like. A fistula can also burrow into the top of the vagina causing faeces to leak from there. Clearly, these are horrifying symptoms for anyone to experience, and they are challenging to treat, so seeking early medical intervention is to be encouraged. It is important to point out that even the most complex fistulas can be dealt with in most cases.

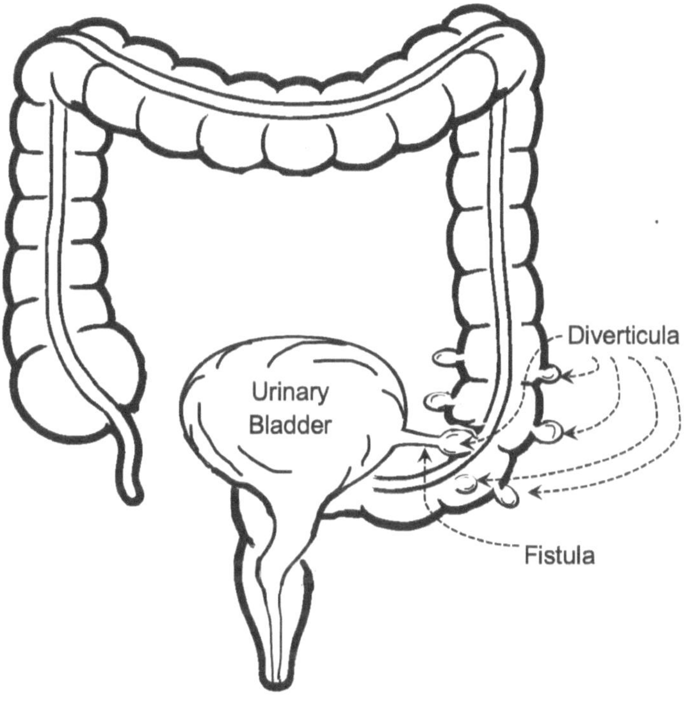

Figure 4. Diverticulum leading to fistula from gut into bladder.

Stricture

Just as a scar on the hand can contract and become tight, the same thing can happen in the colon. Recurrent episodes of diverticulitis cause some scarring in the gut, and the shrinking of this scar may lead to a *stricture*—a narrowed area. This will lead to further pressure rises upstream increasing the likelihood of further problems in diverticula in that area. The stricture will impact the size of faeces that can pass through, and symptoms will include constipation, passing ever-smaller faeces, nausea, vomiting, cramping abdominal pain and abdominal swelling. With an attack, one can commonly experience *tenesmus,* a sense of incomplete emptying, or the feeling of a constant need to defecate. This can also be associated with a cancer or other tumour in the rectum or anus.

Bleeding

Remember our anatomy lesson? It is between the colonic muscle bands that diverticula form, right where arteries penetrate the colon wall. Well, if a pouch gets inflamed and sticks to an adjacent artery, the artery can bleed into the colon, leading to bright red blood loss via the anus. This can sometimes be so extreme that it leads to shock and is a major medical emergency. As blood pressure drops, bleeding might stop and although it might start up again after medical treatment, sometimes it will not recur.

Although each of these may never occur, each time one does the likelihood of a subsequent complication increases. Sooner or later, the doctors may suggest that a preemptive strike to remove diseased bowel is called for. Certainly, any such complication should inspire patients to take the disease seriously and make some changes to do everything they can to prevent diverticulitis flaring up.

4

The Doctor's Finger Is In

Dr. Google

So, you have a gut feeling – and not a good one – that something is wrong. Off you go to the doctor. Right? Hopefully, but that's often not what people do. Nowadays people consult Dr. Google. The last time we checked, Dr. G does not have a medical degree—although our Dr. G does! You see, there is a way of thinking, of processing information, which can lead to the most efficient diagnosis and treatment: a doctor hears you describe your medical history and your symptoms, performs an examination and orders carefully selected investigations based on your history and physical findings. While a physician's approach is not without flaw, it tends to be safer and kinder than searching online, which

> It's not just Dr. Google now. We've got a bunch of AIs answering peoples' questions. Maybe they are accurate. Maybe they are hallucinating. Be very careful as we all sort out how to use these AIs.

can provide misleading, worrying and downright incorrect information. And remember, because the internet uses algorithms, when you enter a set of symptoms you may be guided to a result that has more to do with your search history than what is going on inside. Additionally, unlike physicians, Dr. Google does not particularly care about your privacy. Anything you type in will become part of your profile, shared with those who wish to market you *stuff*. And when it comes to marketing medical or health *stuff* on the internet, that stuff is often junk.

There are other challenges nowadays: in the UK, limited resources in our stretched National Health Service might constrain one's access to a timely appointment. In the USA, cost may be a factor (whether insured or not) and, for better or worse, many American practices use non-physician medical practitioners, not just to triage care, but to provide care in entirety.

> Non-physician practitioners undertake far less formal medical education and training than physicians do. But an experienced nurse practitioner or physician's assistant may well be a better provider of care for you than an inexperienced new doctor.

Advocacy

It is therefore important if you have diverticulosis (or any condition) to advocate for yourself. To optimize a medical clinic visit, try going to the appointment with notes tabulating your symptoms, how long they have been present, what is the nature of any pain and how symptoms are exacerbated by certain things or soothed by others. Do not be afraid to ask your physician questions. It might be worthwhile bringing along a close relative or friend: we know that people often forget what was and was not discussed during a medical consultation. A second set of ears and hands taking written notes is no bad thing. Some people like to record the visit on their smart phone but always ask your doctor's permission first.

If you are not satisfied with the resolution of the consultation, seek a second opinion. No good doctor should ever hesitate to help you find someone else to validate or question what he or she has told you. If one doctor says, "It's nothing serious," but your gut says otherwise, consult another expert. A second opinion can provide clarity, confirm or challenge an initial diagnosis, and offer peace of mind. After all, even Sherlock Holmes never solved a case on intuition alone. Nowadays, you may be able get remote second opinions via video conference with highly experienced physicians.

I introduced John, Nigel and myself as sailors. Well, advocating for yourself and navigating your medical care is like being the captain of your own ship. You're out there on the high seas of jargon and insurance paperwork, steering toward the elusive continent of Diagnosis, island of Treatment and five-star resort of Recovery. The healthcare system, as complex and fragmented as a jigsaw puzzle with missing pieces, often leaves patients feeling like they're a one-legged man in an ass-kicking contest. More than 70% of Americans believe their medical system doesn't meet their needs because of its confusing logistics and inflated costs. This is why advocacy is essential. With this book and other resources, you have a compass, guiding you through stormy waters, ensuring you're heard, understood, and taken seriously.

Being an advocate for yourself means channeling your inner detective. It involves gathering clues, asking questions, and refusing to settle for vague answers. You need to be proactive. Pay attention to one simple fact; this is your medical problem, and you need to understand every element of what is going on.

Together with detailed notes of your symptoms, be sure to document all conversations with medical providers, and at the end of any consultation read the conclusions or recommendations back to the doctor to confirm you understood. This is not about being adversarial; doctors truly want to help, but that requires clear and honest communication between medic and patient. Sometimes the doctors don't do that well and need you to nudge them to communicate completely.

Here is an example of how it can so easily go wrong; a patient comes into clinic saying they have an overly frequent need to have a poop. The clinic secretary records this (wrongly) as *diarrhoea.* Neither the clinic secretary nor the patient knows that diarrhoea is not the same as frequent need to poop. But the clinician moving quickly along finds that the patient is having to go to the toilet 10 times a day and prescribes something to make the stool firmer. However, the patient *didn't have diarrhoea.* Diarrhoea means faeces that has an excessively high-water content. It is separate and different from *frequency of defaecation.* People with diverticulitis can feel the urge to poop frequently—nearly all the time, while not having diarrhoea, and indeed be constipated. A doctor can march down a path that is entirely wrong, and if they do so with an authoritative voice, a patient may just shut up and not push back (so to speak). Be patient with the doctor but don't be that patient who doesn't push back. If something the doctor is saying doesn't make sense, explain that they may have a mistaken assumption, and ask questions.

A Quick Checklist for Advocacy

- **Prepare for Appointments**: Write down your symptoms, questions, and concerns.
- **Take a friend**: Brief them beforehand about why you are seeing the doctor, ask them to bring along a notepad and ensure they understand they are there to encourage and support you.
- **Ask Questions**: Don't be afraid to seek clarity on medical terms or procedures.

- **Request a Second Opinion:** If uncertain, consult another healthcare provider.
- **Document Everything**: Keep a journal of symptoms, treatments, and doctor visits. Doing so makes it so much more efficient for subsequent visits or seeing another doctor.
- **Be Persistent**: Follow up on test results and next steps. Yes, the doctor or hospital should let you know results but after all, if there is a slip-up in the system it is you who will suffer! Let's reiterate this: Don't trust the administrative system. And when it comes to physicians: *trust but verify.*

> Electronic medical records (EMRs) serve some valuable roles but also cause huge problems. In America, EMR's are built for the primary purpose of optimizing billing, and only secondarily attend to documenting medical care for the benefit of the patient. EMR's are cluttered with checkboxes. Sometimes these help physicians remember to ask questions, sometimes they turn a doctor-patient relationship into a doctor-computer relationship. So keep your own notes!

Navigating the healthcare system requires patience, persistence, and a bit of chutzpah. We're thinking about writing a book on this topic. But you are your own best advocate, and with the right tools, you can effectively manage your health and your medical care.

Seeing your doctor

Let's face it, talking to a doctor about your digestive woes can feel as awkward as discussing your teenage diary entries. But when it comes to gut health, it's time to put on your brave pants and get chatty about your poop. Your doctor needs to know what's happening down there to figure out what's really going on. Approach this conversation with confidence and set aside embarrassment, for I assure you, the doctor has heard it all!

Nothing, absolutely nothing, surprises an experienced physician.

The first step in the diagnostic journey is the *History,* which has two components. The first is where you narrate your medical story in your own words, however you feel you need to. This is usually in response to a doctor asking, "What brought you here today?" And while it might be tempting to say, "my sister's car" or "an Uber," please resist the urge – remember, we have heard pretty much every joke there is to tell. And we've told so many bad jokes that we know what bad jokes look like.

Below we will give you some of the elements the doctors most need to hear.

Start by explaining how long these mysterious symptoms have been impacting you and point to exactly where you feel each. Are they a recent development, or have they been hanging around for "a while"? Give your doctor a timeline, because "a while" is a meaningless term. The doctor needs to get a sense of whether they're dealing with an acute concern or a long-term issue.

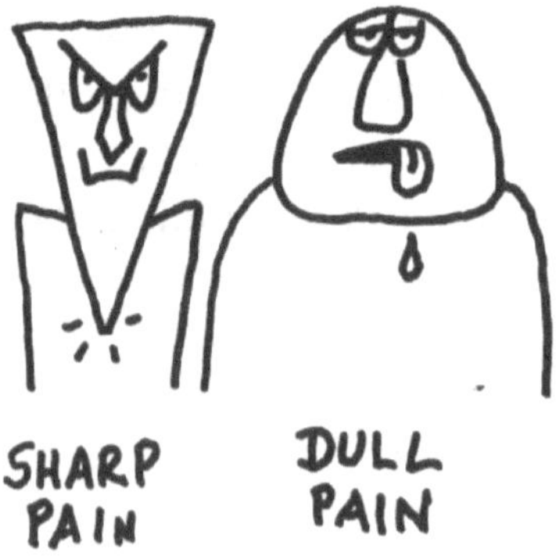

Next, paint a picture of any pain, or the "quality" as we call it (which always struck me as an odd use of the word!) Is it sharp, dull, or somewhere in between? Do the episodes last a few minutes and then fade, or do they linger? How severe is the pain – can you muddle through, or do you need to lie down and scream? The more descriptive you are, the better your doctor can turn your symptoms into a list of potential diagnoses. Don't shy away from spilling the beans on what makes things worse. Even beans. Maybe it's that spicy taco you just couldn't resist or, if you are an anxious type, the stress of remembering your neighbor's cat's birthday. Identifying these triggers gives your doctor a clue about what might be exacerbating your condition.

On the flip side, share any tricks that bring relief. Maybe lying down helps, or perhaps a cup of chamomile tea does the trick. These anecdotes are breadcrumbs leading to the right diagnosis. And while you're at it, don't forget your digestive history. Have you danced this dance before? Any past intestinal escapades your doctor should know about? Include anything else you might have noticed when the symptoms pay you an uninvited visit.

Next up your doctor will go a little bit legal eagle on you and ask questions about specific aspects of your health. Frankly it is a worthwhile project to carefully document this and have a copy ready at hand and with a loved one should the need arise. To make it easier, we have a form in Appendix I for you to use but broadly speaking, this is how it will go:

Family history: Age of parents and first-degree relatives, diseases and causes of death. Has anyone in your biologically related family had similar medical problems to yours? I once saw a patient with abdominal pain, and the clue was that his father and brother also had similar pain. Turned out to be a rare disease called *porphyria* and I would never have thought of this were it not for the family history.

Social history: Do you smoke, drink, use recreational drugs? Please tell the truth – we were always told that a man will admit to smoking 10 cigarettes a day, his wife will say 40 and the truth lies somewhere in between. They will ask about employment, travel, even pets. If that sounds odd, please know that there are several diseases that can be transferred from pets to humans; we are not just being nosy. And if you consume a specific diet or avoid certain foods, please tell your doctor as all of this may be relevant and can lead to diagnoses other than diverticulosis.

Previous medical history: This will be divided into medical and surgical and each needs to include what happened, when it happened, who looked after you, and is there ongoing treatment or planned follow up. You will need to provide a list of medications taken, whether prescription, over the counter or alternative medicines (some of which can interfere with prescription drugs or be harmful). Include any allergies to food or drugs – people with a seafood allergy may have a negative reaction to an agent used in certain medical imaging studies – make sure you tell your physician. Nowadays the term "allergy" is bandied about quite freely and many reactions to food, for instance, are not true allergies – make sure you are specific and precise as to what happens when you take a given substance or food.

Systems review: Your doctor will now go through each of the body systems asking very targeted leading questions; it is imperative you answer these fully and accurately as your responses will guide what your doctor may be looking for and what tests might be ordered. They may start with four general questions:

i. How is your appetite?

ii. What is your weight doing? Any recent unplanned weight loss or unexpected gain?

iii. Are you feeling generally well or unwell?

iv. What are your energy levels?

Other questions will target body systems and will include the following, although this list is by no means exhaustive:

Cardiovascular: Chest pain, palpitations, pain in legs when walking, fingers or toes get cold and/or change colour

Respiratory: difficulty breathing, cough and whether it is productive, breathlessness at rest, exercise, lying flat or during the night,

Central nervous: headache, eyesight or hearing abnormalities or loss, change in sense of taste or smell, areas of weakness or strange sensation, any tremors, loss of consciousness or seizures

Gastrointestinal: dry mouth, difficulty swallowing, heartburn, nausea or vomiting, change in frequency and nature of bowel motions, presence of blood or mucus in faeces

Genitourinary: change in frequency of passing urine during day and night, difficulty urinating, change in colour or smell, pain. Normal pregnancy is not a disease of course, but it's important for the doctor to know if you are pregnant.

Skin: Rashes, itching, colour, changes in hair or nails

Musculoskeletal: aches or pains, issues with joint movement or rigidity

Physical examination

Equipped with your story, the doc will now want to examine you. If you have any concerns about your sense of comfort, remember it is your right to ask for there to be a chaperone present. You will likely be asked to don a highly fashionable gown with your sit-upon exposed for the world (or at least your doctor) to see. And no, we physicians have no idea why the gowns are designed the way they are. They've been that way for 100 years. We figure it's part of the patriarchy, or some such.

Truly, those gowns are perfect for getting a colonoscopy (to be discussed later). But for the physical exam, they are rather silly.

First, there will be measurements of your height and weight so an estimate of body mass index (BMI) can be made. In other words, is your weight healthy, or are you fat enough that you have increased risk for various diseases, or thin enough to raise concerns about malnutrition or chronic illness? This is done in context: one can have a "healthy" BMI but demonstrate poor muscle mass and signs of unwanted weight loss. You can calculate your BMI either using an online calculator like the one provided by the NHS https://www.nhs.uk/health-assessment-tools/calculate-your-body-mass-index/calculate-bmi-for-adults or from the US Centers for Disease Control https://www.cdc.gov/bmi/adult-calculator/index.html. Or if you are a mathematical whizz, divide your weight by height squared (in metric measurements). So, if you weigh 70kg and are 1.75 metres tall, first multiple 1.75 x 1.75 which equals 3.0625. Then divide 70 by 3.0625 which yields a healthy BMI of 22.86.

> If you are an American, or an old-fashioned Brit, convert your weight and height into metric before doing the math. Alternatively, divide your weight in pounds by your height in inches squared, then multiply by 703!

Generally speaking:

- BMI less than 18.5 implies being underweight
- 18.5 – 25 healthy weight
- 25 – 30 overweight

Above 30 is considered obese. And then there are those at a BMI of 40 or above who are considered seriously, or *morbidly* obese. *Morbid* means different things to different physicians, but to the three of us it means that the obesity is not just a risk for a disease but is a disease itself.

BMI is a useful tool, but there are caveats; very athletic folks might have a number that puts them in the overweight category because muscle is heavier than fat. When pregnant, BMI is not a sensible tool for obvious reasons. For certain folk, disease and operative outcome risks are higher with an elevated BMI than other folks. For those under age 18, different charts are used, but in the context of diverticulosis—which is vanishingly rarely a pediatric illness—this is not relevant

Next up, the doctor will do some general checks. Do you look anaemic or jaundiced? Are you well proportioned? Do you seem able to clearly understand what is going on? They will then check all the other systems to include blood pressure, pulse, checking your heart and lungs.

You might think, "I came to the doctor with a sore belly and the idiot wanted to check my chest, ears, eyes and even my nails!" Please know that they are usually doing these checks to firstly ensure there is nothing else going on, and secondly to make a general health assessment that will inform a plan of action once the diagnosis is made. And some of the seemingly bonkers stuff? Well, there is method in the madness. For instance, in Crohn's disease, which can mimic diverticulitis, one can get signs in the eye like redness called *episcleritis* (there it is again – "-itis") and changes in the fingernail shape called *clubbing*. And there are many more of these esoteric signs that doctors know about and try to catch. That is why some of the more masochistic doctors love watching medical shows like *House*......or ER ("errrr" as we pronounce it) just so we can scream at the TV when they get it wrong.

Checking out your abdomen may start with a peek into your mouth to smell your breath, check teeth, gums and the other membranes. One rare but very nasty sequel of diverticulitis (and bowel cancer) is where inflamed transverse colon sticks to and burrows into the bottom of the stomach. This fistula allows faeces to dwell in the stomach causing a particular kind of foul breath. We are also checking for ulcers and other signs that might indicate the colon issue is inflammatory bowel disease like Crohn's or ulcerative colitis – a topic for a future book.

Soon enough the focus at long last will be on your belly. There are four phases of this focus, and a wee surprise!

i. *Inspection:* we surgeons look at the abdomen from the foot of the bed and traditionally examine from the right side of the bed. We are looking for discoloration of the skin, movement with breathing, any obvious swellings or distension and scars from prior operations or interventions. There are some specific visible signs of ongoing intraabdominal trouble. One example is Cullen's sign, where there are bruises around the belly button despite no injury there. It means something pretty bad is going on in the belly. In circumstances where there is generalized inflammation, the patient may well be immobile.

> On the other side of the Atlantic, physicians may stand on the left. In Australia, they stand upside down.

ii. *Percussion:* this means, as the name suggests, to use your body (and in this case your belly) as a drum set. By tapping in various areas, we can ascertain whether what should sound hollow does, in fact, sound hollow. There are also some cool tricks like checking for a "thrill." Rather than being utterly inappropriate, this is where one taps one flank and feels for vibrations on the other side, an indication of fluid inside the belly cavity in places where it shouldn't be.

iii. *Palpation:* this means to feel, and is performed with the physician's hands, area by area, seeking any masses, checking the organs (including liver and spleen) and ascertaining any areas of tenderness. If one presses on the left side of the belly and pain is felt on the right, this suggests inflammation around the appendix (Rovsing's sign). And if pain is generalized (all over the belly), it implies peritonitis (a bad thing): the patient will guard their belly wall against the doctor's hands, move little and tense their abdominal muscles. If the doctor presses down, it will be tender, but on releasing pres-

> We love to give old dead surgeons credit. Probably because Jonathan will someday be an old dead surgeon.

sure, the pain is even worse, so-called rebound tenderness, or Blumberg's sign.

iv. *Auscultation:* is where we listen to the abdomen with a stethoscope and characterize the nature, frequency and volume of gut sounds. For instance, if high-pitched and frequent, that may imply a bowel obstruction: silence suggests ileus, which is when the guts shut down because of inflammation or metabolic problems that can occur with illness, dehydration, vomiting, or post-operatively. We can also hear sounds that can lead to a diagnosis of a diseased major blood vessel that can be life-threatening.

v. *Wee surprise:* Ever watched the Chevy Chase movie *Fletch*, where he visits a doctor, has a rectal exam and sings Moon River? Well, that's next up, if you will forgive the pun as your doctor dons a rubber glove and has you assume the position on your left side. Singing Moon River or other tunes is not obligatory but will doubtless make your doctor's day. The doctor is feeling for masses and areas of tenderness and will chemically check for hidden (occult) stool blood on their gloved finger after the exam is complete. It's not a pleasant way to spend a minute, but as we were taught, if the doctor doesn't put their finger in it, they will put their foot in it by missing something important!

> This is called a digital rectal exam. Digital means the doctor's finger (digit), not a computer program.

> In medical school we are taught there are only two reasons not to perform a rectal exam: 1) no finger. 2) No rectum. For better or worse, most doctors ignore that lesson. But when it comes to diagnosing intestinal disease, a rectal exam is needed.

So, what have we learned?

Understanding medical terminology is like learning a new language—except there's no app for that. When your doctor starts speaking Latin and you don't have a clue what he's talking about, don't hesitate to say *"Sua mihi omnia Graeca"* meaning "It's all Greek to me." It's important to understand what's being said, so there's no shame in asking for clarifications. If your doctor mentions something that sounds like a Harry Potter spell, make sure you get a translation. You're there to get answers, not to earn a degree in medicine. Doctors sometimes forget not everyone misspent their youth boning up on bones with weird names, so remind them gently that you *left your stethoscope at home*.

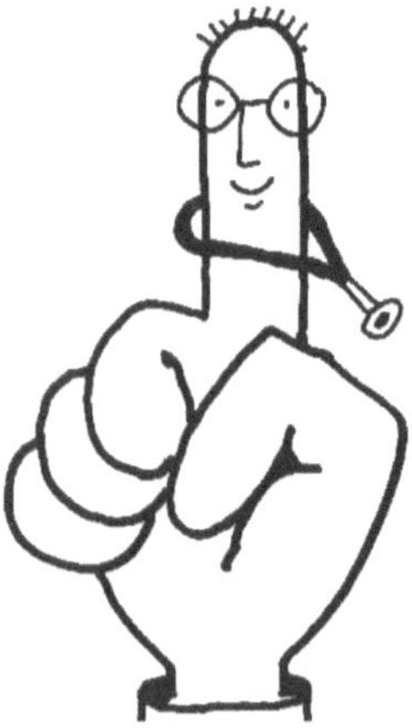

Keeping track of your symptoms over time is as important as balancing your bank cheque book used to be back when there were cheque books. So, keep a journal and document what transpired at this consultation then check that your interpretation gels with the doctor's.

As you wrap up this chapter, remember that open dialogue with your doctor is the key to unlocking the mysteries of your gut. With a bit of preparation and a dash of humor, you can transform the doctor's office from a place of dread into a space of understanding. Now, with a clearer sense of communication, you're set to explore the next chapter's insights on medical tests and what to expect on your journey to better health.

5

Scan and Deliver

The Colonoscopy Inuendo

Introduction

You know about the medical student who stayed up all night studying for her blood test? Or the one about the blood donor who went out with a nurse, but they had to end it when she discovered he wasn't her type? Having needles, or other things stuck into you is never fun, but it may be a key step on the path to a treatment plan, solving your current problem and avoiding future issues.

The tests your doctor recommends will be driven by the history and physical examination we set out in Chapter 4 and can be divided into those that address the problem at hand – or up your tailpipe – and those that help define your general health so that the right treatment can be delivered. The term "doctor's order" is often used, but misinterpreted. The *order* in question is to the lab or facility that will perform the analysis. You as the patient are *not being ordered to do anything*. We physicians just make recommendations. Take time to find out what each test is, why it is being done, how it will impact your outcome and when you should expect results.

And in the USA particularly, you should certainly ask how much it will cost. Doctors never know the answer to that simple question but asking it just might start another revolution.

Tests specifically for diverticulosis

The purpose here is to confirm whether diverticulosis is indeed the underlying diagnosis and then to define which areas of the colon are affected, how many diverticula are having a get together inside your belly, and are there any signs of ongoing inflammation, narrowing or fistula. We shall reserve for Chapter 9 a discussion about tests that might take place during an acute episode of diverticulitis.

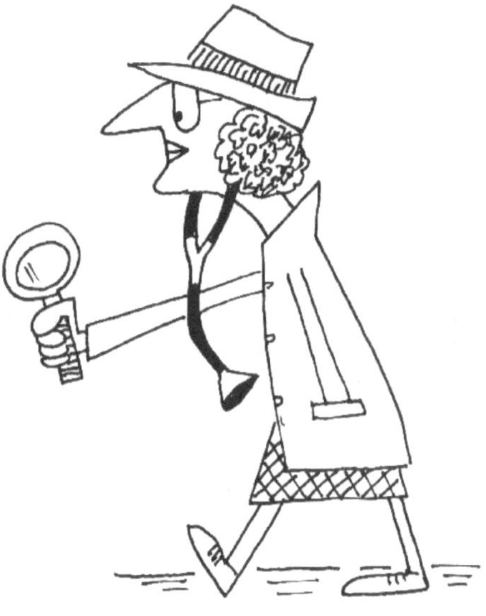

Plain abdominal x rays: These are the simple grayscale images you see on TV, the classic "x-ray." And they are generally of little use in the evaluation of diverticulosis. All one might see is some faeces loading up the colon, and that information can be gleaned from talking to the patient, palpating the abdomen and doing the digital rectal examination we talked about earlier. In these days of "protocol-driven medicine" some insurance companies or other payors demand x-rays be performed first as they are supposedly cheaper, but this is a nonsense and is a waste of time and resources and exposes you to unnecessary radiation. Unless the doctor explains their need for a plain abdominal x-ray, just say no.

Barium enema: Any sentence that contains the word "enema" isn't going to go down well. Or up well. Barium enemas are rarely done nowadays other than in resource-constrained areas of the world that do not have CAT scans (see below). Basically, a tube is inserted into the anus and a paste squeezed in that contains barium (a thick, white, substance that shows up on x-rays). If diverticulosis is present, one sees little round dots alongside the tube of the colon.

CAT scan (or CT scan): This test requires one to lie on a sliding table and pop in and out of a large metal doughnut in which you are the jam. Hundreds of images of your body are shot from all axes or angles and reassembled by a computer into a model of your insides viewed as either horizontal or vertical slices through the belly. The name stands for **C**omputer **A**xial **T**omography, and because it uses x-ray radiation, the radiographer (a qualified technician who looks after you) should place a lead shield over your neck and groin to protect thyroid and testicles. For women the ovaries cannot be shielded as they are deep in the pelvis where we need to see. The scan may be done after you drink a fluid called *contrast* that shows up as dense white in your bowel and better allows doctors to see the outlines. Gas, on the other hand, appears black. Additionally, a different contrast formulation may be injected intravenously to show where the blood vessels are that may be near inflamed diverticula. Ask to see the pictures and have them explained to you – the images are pretty cool, and remember, knowledge is power!

Colonoscopy: This is the gold standard for diagnosing problems inside the colon. We use a flexible snake-like device, around 1.25cm across (around ½ inch) and about a meter (3 feet) long. At the end that goes inside your bottom, there is a silicon chip camera that sends video images to a screen viewed by the operator, usually a gastroenterologist or surgeon, but in some countries, specialist nurses now do this. The tip can be moved left, right, up or down via rotating knobs controlled by the person controlling the device. This *colonoscopist* can also twist the scope and advance it further in. The end also has a bright light and there are channels that allow air to be pumped in to inflate the colon, fluid to be squirted in to move debris out the way, suction to vacuum excess air, liquid and debris, and a *working channel* that allows the doctor to thread long instruments into the colon to take biopsies or do other magic tricks.... although no rabbits appear from this particular hole.

Preparing for the test usually requires a low residue diet for a few days (we'll explain low residue soon), clear fluid diet for at least one day and then a "bowel prep" the evening before. Ask your doctor about what medications you should avoid in the days leading up to your test, such as low-dose aspirin for heart problems or pain relievers like ibuprofen. If a biopsy is required, these drugs can make bleeding worse.

People love to "horribilise" colonoscopy and the prep, but having had a few myself, I can attest to it not being that bad.... not how I would choose to spend a morning, but not that bad. The prep you need to drink either comes as a fluid or a powder to mix with water. Follow the instructions precisely and put the prep in a cold fridge, it is easier to drink that way. You can make your life better by truly avoiding solid foods for a couple of days. Chicken broth and herb teas are fine and make for an easier prep experience. You will want to keep a toilet close at hand, or close to bum, while undergoing the prep. Take a book, a comfy pillow and take a big supply of cold water. For each glass of prep you chug down, drink some water. Yes, the prep can taste foul, but if you drink it quickly and wash it down with water, it is not intolerable. The prep works by sucking fluid out your blood stream and into the colon tube thereby flushing out all bits and pieces of poop. My old joke was that if you think the bottom has dropped out of your world because you need to have a colonoscopy, drink the bowel prep and feel the world drop out your bottom. Because your tail end will be mimicking the nozzle of a Saturn Five rocket, I always recommend staying ahead of the game and smearing some Vaseline on the area in question ahead of the first jet to prevent any soreness. And by the way, the rocket analogy during the prep is apt. Another good analogy is your bum will mimic a firehose.

You will basically have a Niagara Falls version of diarrhoea for a few hours. You must finish enough of the prep until it comes out from your tailpipe totally clear, water in water out. That way the doctor's view will not be impeded by debris on the bowel wall. There are a variety of different prep regimes so be sure to follow what you are given to the letter; some require you to drink more on the day of the procedure.

Make sure someone will take you to the test, or collect you after the test, as the team will have sedated you for the procedure. When you enter the colonoscopy room, they will have you wear that stylish gown with your arse hanging in the breeze. This time, that gown makes sense. With an IV set up to administer fluids, you will lie on your left side and some magic medicine will be given to you to help you slip off to sleep.

While you are in the Land of Nod, the doctor steers the scope up your rectum, taking time to turn back on itself to get a turd's eye view of the inside of the anus. Then it's back to the task at hand, a straight trip up the rectum and then a series of twists and turns through the sigmoid with no clear tunnel obvious followed by the straight shot up the descending colon. On reaching the left rib cage, the colon turns right under the spleen and the tunnel diameter is minimized as a result. The transverse colon is easily identified as it looks like a triangle, then it's a quick left turn under the liver and drop down into the caecum, a quick visit into the small bowel and say *Hi* to the appendix. Along the way photos will be snapped. After all, when you go on a trip surely you take pictures? If one sees round black holes off to the side that is a sure sign of diverticulosis, each being an entry point into a diverticulum, Figure 5 gives some idea what it looks like. We also check for narrowed or inflamed areas and anything else that does not look right.

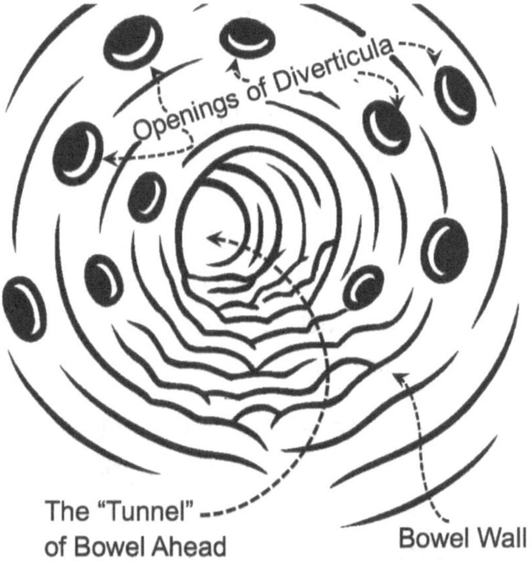

Figure 5. Diverticula from the endoscopist's point of view

The next thing you know, you will awaken and be given the results by the doctor and shown some of the travel photos from the trip. You can hang them up on your refrigerator with magnets.

After telling you what was found, the doctor should advise that some air was blown up your colon and will doubtless find its way out over the next few hours. Nothing to be concerned about. Colonoscopy is a common and safe procedure, but complications can occur, although rarely, the most serious of which is a tear or perforation of the bowel or bleeding from a biopsy. You will be advised what to look out for, but if symptoms occur, even days later, It is critically important that you head back to hospital to be evaluated.

Capsule endoscopy: Two very smart chaps, scientist Gavriel Iddan and gastroenterologist Eitan Scapa dreamed up the idea of an endoscope you could swallow. They created a pill-sized camera—brilliantly called the Pillcam—that would send photos back to the outside world as it made its journey from mouth to anus. It is quite useful to address problems in the upper gut and the small intestine where scopes cannot travel, but less so for diverticulosis where it is rarely used other than for research purposes.

Virtual colonoscopy: This is where a CAT scan is used leveraging 3D computer graphics and clever software to image what is going on inside the colon without the need for a colonoscope to come within a mile of your derrière or anaesthesia in your veins. However, if one sees an abnormality that requires a biopsy, a true endoscopy is required. Although patients do find it more acceptable than the scope (I wonder why?), its optimum place in clinical practice is still being evaluated.

General medical tests

While some blood tests may be affected by the presence of diverticulitis, the following are done to see what is going on more generally, to ascertain the impact of the disease on your health and to risk stratify should surgical intervention prove necessary.

Blood tests:

CBC/FBC: the complete or full blood count measures multiple blood parameters. It can help assess oxygen carrying capacity, if there has been any blood loss or anaemia from chronic disease, whether your white blood cells are normal or suggestive of infection, and some perspectives on blood clotting.

U&E (Urea and Electrolytes or Metabolic Panel): this blood test measures how the kidneys are performing both in terms of general health and if various minerals are in balance.

LFTs: Liver Function Tests are a misnomer in that they are better described as liver dysfunction tests. They are a good marker of whether the liver is inflamed. Additional blood tests that assess blood protein levels and other parameters of good health can also inform about liver function.

Clotting studies: as the name suggests, these can tell us if your blood is properly able to stop bleeding should the need arise.

Inflammatory markers: ESR measures how cells in a column of blood settle in a tube, the higher the number, the higher the indication that inflammation is active. One can also measure CRP, a protein that is a sensitive marker of inflammation, but tells little to nothing about where that inflammation may be.

Tumour markers: given the symptoms of diverticulosis might also raise the concern of colon cancer, the doctor may deem it shrewd to look for some chemicals in the blood that are found when there is a cancer lurking.

X-rays: While plain films of the abdomen are of little value, a chest x-ray is a useful tool prior to many medical interventions (surgery, etc.), because it can reveal covert lung or heart disease. It is a common test on admission to hospital.

ECG: The electrocardiogram is a way of gaining a window into how the heart is working. You see, in that key organ there are highly orchestrated electrical waves that travel around the muscle via a type of biologic wiring called the Bundle of His after electrical energy has been generated by two little biologic powerplants. An ECG provides us with a piece of paper that looks at the heart from twelve different perspectives and allows us to diagnose

> In the US, EKG is used although "K" appears nowhere in the name, it is a throwback to the German origin of the phrase. In Britain we add unnecessary letters to words, so who are we to critique our friends across the pond?

prior "silent" heart attacks, dodgy rhythms and sometimes even heart attacks threatening to happen.

Pulmonary function tests: If surgery is required it may prove judicious for the anaesthetist to check lung function by having you blow into a special measuring device. Whenever I tried to convince a smoker to give up – a very tough ask – one technique that I found worked was to show them what a normal test looked like then have them do it. There was an uncomfortable moment, occasionally an insult directed at me for tricking them, but often, the colour would drain from their face and the cigarette packet would be thrown away there and then.

Results

Often, results are posted onto a computerized patient portal to which you have access over the internet. However, understanding test reports can be like reading a novel in a foreign language. The key is in the summary and recommendations section, where the doctor will lay out what the findings mean for you. If there is no simple description, please do not google the words as the context may be misunderstood. A colon polyp can be anything from an irrelevance to a malignant tumour. If you do not understand something, be sure to seek rapid clarification so your anxiety does not ramp up. Avoid the tragedy of developing serious anxiety in the wake of a misunderstood, harmless diagnosis!

> Patients are starting to load their medical results into AI to help them understand them. If you choose that route, please don't panic if the AI says something you don't want to hear. Just call your doctor. Remember, AIs can and do hallucinate.

With the knowledge of basic medical tests in hand, we'll soon shift focus to the nitty-gritty of diet and lifestyle changes, where the rubber meets the road in managing these conditions and preventing *-osis* from becoming *-itis*!

6

The Gut Whisperer

Dr. John Hunt's Personal Experiences with Diverticulosis and Diverticulitis

You've just been handed the diagnosis, and now it's time to figure out how to deal with it. There is much you can do to keep yourself flatulating wisely and safely. With a bit of knowledge, you can become your own gut whisperer, learning the subtle cues and signals your digestive system sends before it goes pit bull on your ass. Yes, ass, I am an American so the heck with arse! The material in this chapter emphasizes what has gone before, and it is doubtless repeated and expanded upon later in the book. Repetition helps to get the stuff to sink in so that the poop can get out effortlessly.

Triggers and avoidance tactics

Hi, this is Dr. John Hunt here and I have written this section of the book. Why? Well, because I am the proud owner of a bunch of diverticula in my colon and I also have some novel views on the medical system that I use to help understand how things work and don't work for my patients. Including me. Here's some of it.

I define *health care* as those things you do to maintain your own health. Health care is therefore mostly free, requires no administrators, no physicians, no hospitals and no procedures. Health care (by my definition) consists of four (and a half) components:

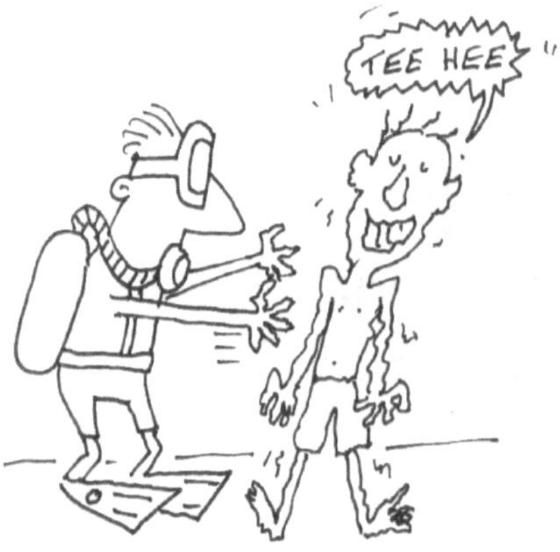

DIVER-TICKLE-YA

1. **Nutrition that is appropriate for you,**
2. **Exercise/general fitness,**
3. **Good sleep, and**
4. **Stress moderation.**

4½. The half component isn't quite free and involves a bit of expertise: selected vaccinations.

Together, these four (and a half) components of health care keep you healthy, most of the time. But sometimes even your best health care efforts fail. And that's when medical care comes in.

Medical care (again by your colon commentator's preferred definition) is what you need when your health care efforts have *not* kept you healthy. Medical care involves doctors and other clinicians, medications, technology and other interventions to return you to health.

Caring for your health is a good way to limit your need for medical care and the expenses associated with it. This is particularly true for people with diverticulosis. It turns out that simply (or not so simply) living more healthily is the best thing you can do to live well with diverticulosis, therefore minimizing episodes of diverticulitis and risks of needing surgery. Frankly, if everyone paid more attention to health care, they would have to pay less attention to medical care. And less money.

Nutrition and your choice of foods

Everybody's different. Every *body's* different. Some foods cause gas in one person and not another person. Some people will get gas with some fibre, yet not other fibres. Therefore, your food choices and medication choices will need to be individualized based on what you learn about yourself.

Your gut may tolerate foods that the guts of other people with diverticulosis and diverticulitis can't tolerate. And vice versa. So, you can read all the dietary recommendations on the planet—recommendations that may be well advised for Average Joe—but that turn out not to be well advised for you at all. Given that you most certainly are not the Average Joe, how can you sort out what you should eat and not eat?

It's not that hard to do but takes some time and thought. Pay attention to the food you eat, and the symptoms that arise in the 1-24 hours after eating it. Write this info down in a diary or type it into your notes on a phone, because brain memory is unreliable while cloud memory is forever. Sure, if you take notes on your phone, anthropology PhD students 500 years from now will be able to write their theses on your bowel habits (if that's their thing). But you'll be long dead by then and won't care. Or perhaps you might appreciate the fame. So today, keeping good track for a month or two can help you for the rest of your life. Start making notes on which foods, and other things, adversely affect how your gut feels.

Let's start with a nutshell that serves as an example of how I think about triggers of my own diverticulitis. I can't eat peanuts or walnuts without paying a price, but I can wolf down almonds and cashews. But you are neither me nor the Average Joe, so what one bowel autobiographer and another Average Joe can and cannot eat is irrelevant to you.

Doctors used to tell patients with diverticulosis not to eat nuts. Then they did some research studies and proved that nuts don't cause problems for diverticulosis and even started recommending nuts for their fibre content. Go figure: one day we say this, then we say that. Importantly, you weren't enrolled in the study, and any such study is always looking at averages and probabilities. No study in which you don't participate yourself is going to be able to tell *you* if nuts are a problem for *you* or not.

So, instead, pay attention to yourself. If you already know that your gut raises a stink when you eat nuts, then, by all means, stop eating nuts! It may be that some nuts cause you problems and others don't. Some people seem sensitive only to tree nuts, and not ground nuts (peanuts live underground, not dangling from trees). Others, of course, suffer from peanuts. Or you may totally tolerate all nuts, in which case, just pay attention, and don't outright ban them. And if unsure, put your nuts on the back burner.

Foods that cause you gas should be minimized, because gas in your gut can balloon out the diverticula. By your age, you probably have a reasonable concept of what causes you worse bouts of gas, but if not, start paying heed and keeping a diary for a while and you will soon sort it out. Maybe you can turn the diary into a novel, or perhaps a screenplay.

If you are intolerant of any foods, you may also have inflammatory responses to those foods. Inflammation in a diverticulum turns it into diverticulitis. (Remember, "-itis" means "inflammation"). Food allergies are one cause of inflammation.

If you think you may have food allergies, then you can be tested. Although tests are helpful, they need to be interpreted with great caution. First, there are oodles of false positives, meaning a test may say you have a problem but be entirely wrong. Then there are false negative results when the test is reported as negative, but you have the problem. So, when it comes to food allergy testing, only do so under the guidance of a wise allergist who can help you interpret the results. We do not recommend seeing an ENT (otolaryngologist) or chiropractic doctor for your allergy testing, because while they are good at what they do best, allergy *isn't* what they do best. You can start with a family practitioner but consider seeing an allergist before cutting foods out of your diet based on any lab test.

Importantly, specific foods can cause problems for you whether or not you are allergic to them. As an example, some people with diverticulosis have problems with sesame seeds and others with dairy, even when allergy tests or other medical tests don't raise flags. Other people will have immunologic responses to egg that don't show up in routinely available allergy tests, or indeed in any tests. Which brings us back to the test that really matters, which is how your gut responds to foods you eat. You don't need expensive tests if every time you eat eggs you get diarrhoea. To figure it out, you just need your gut and your brain.

Non-food triggers

Your nervous system has various parts, one big component of which is the autonomic system that does stuff you need to live, moderating how your heart beats and gut works for instance. The autonomic system is, in turn, divided into two parts, the *parasympathetic* which manages digestion, relaxation and sex—the good happy stuff. Then there is the *sympathetic nervous system,* which is your "fight or flight" mechanism preparing you for challenging situations, keeping you alive so you can later enjoy the happy stuff. When you are under threat and most need your sympathetic nervous system to be active, digestion is the last thing on your brain's mind.

Stress activates your sympathetic nervous system, releasing hormones that cause intestinal spasms and worsen symptoms. These can change the internal pressure of the gut and irritate diverticulosis. So, minimizing stresses in your life that you know cause your gut to feel like crap is eminently sensible and is based in medical fact. The best strategy is to eliminate or at least mitigate stress, but if you cannot do that, try to find ways to manage it, like yoga or meditation (discussed in chapter 11), which can help your gut as well as your mind.

Stress is an issue, but when it comes to diverticulosis, the elephant poop in the room is *constipation*. This is such an important issue that we present it several times in this book. Constipation is the big enemy of your gut health, and indeed your entire health. Put a big focus on avoiding constipation.

Words matter (and especially so in medicine) which is why it is critical to ensure we know what each word means. Constipation is when one has difficulty passing a bowel motion and the faeces may be harder than usual.

Constipation can be precipitated by traveling, or dehydration, or dehydration *from* traveling, or from dehydration from delaying pooping to avoid using public toilets, or from certain medications such as pain medications, especially opiates, antihistamines, anticholinergics, new migraine drugs and many others. Sometimes there is no evident cause, and your digestive system decides to take a vacation without telling you. Women also report changes in gut behavior at various times in their menstrual cycle. But whatever the cause, when the gut slows down, pressure builds up, and your diverticula start plotting mischief.

Avoiding constipation involves staying hydrated (always) and, for most people, eating a high-fibre diet. Your gut loves routine, so aim for regular mealtimes and bathroom breaks to avoid any unplanned gut surprises. Importantly, when you need to go, *go*!

If you must take constipating medications, make damn sure you do all that you can to keep your gut flowing. Whatever tricks to avoid constipation that you find work for you, use them when you take such meds.

As mentioned, traveling can be a problem. Whether it's a long flight or a road trip, being away from your routine can lead to dehydration. When flying as passenger (or pilot!) avoid alcohol as it dehydrates one at any time and in the "thin" atmosphere of an aircraft this effect is magnified. Dehydration leads to constipation, which is likely one of the worse triggers of flare-ups of your disease. For those who take motion sickness pills, they can lead to constipation. To keep things running smoothly, plan with known safe foods, and *stay hydrated*. And don't forget fibre-rich snacks to keep your digestive system on track.

Fibre always needs to be taken with large amounts of water, because that is how fibre works. Fibre is, by definition, indigestible. Fibre's purpose is to hold water inside the gut, which helps to prevent constipation. But if you are one of those who can't tolerate fibre without getting gassy, there are other ways to keep things moving.

> The laxatives most people think of are stimulants in pill form like senna that inspire your gut nerves to fire and can cause cramping and a very sudden urge to poop. These are not recommended if you have diverticulosis as they may induce higher pressures inside the gut.

Other types of laxatives are osmotic agents that keep water in the bowel and can even pull water into the colon from the blood. There are several of these that have been in use for decades. One such medications is *polyethylene glycol*, or "PEG." There are many brands available. We have made a commitment to not "sell" any particular product, but it would be churlish not to mention that I favor any brand or generic of PEG as the magic bullet for my own gut, because regular fibre makes your faithful farting doctor's gut sound—and feel—like a 7th grade orchestra. PEG comes as a powder one mixes with water, rather like fibre preparations, and is gentle. Incidentally, PEG is also the most common means of cleaning out the bowel ahead of a colonoscopy as described in Chapter 5. It is derived from *ethylene glycol*, the main ingredient in antifreeze for car radiators. I find it amusing to consider my bowels won't ice over in winter. Our good Professor Sackier likes to recommend another such medication, dioctyl sodium sulfosuccinate, not because it is better, but just because he likes saying it.

Again, avoiding constipation is probably the most important key for you to prevent diverticulitis flare-ups. Maintaining a high-fibre diet and/or using daily PEG will help most people avoid constipation and have added benefits of improving bowel function and possibly reducing the risk of colon cancer too. So, likely a win-win.

BUT, and this is another big butt, conventional wisdom states that if you have active diverticulitis, many physicians recommend a "low residue" diet until the diverticulitis settles down. This will be discussed further shortly.

Seek balance by finding ways to enjoy your favorite foods in moderation, avoiding foods you know cause you problems, and prioritizing those that keep your gut happy.

To identify personal triggers of diverticular symptoms, do start by keeping a detailed food and symptom diary, documenting what you eat, how you feel, and any patterns that emerge. This can help you pinpoint what might be causing flare-ups, whether it's spicy curry or the stress induced by having a fight with your spouse. So, if you feel a fracas coming on and exotic food is not a trigger, avoid the argument and head out for an Indian meal. This detective work can help you make informed choices that keep your gut on an even keel. Practicing stress management techniques daily can also ward off unwanted episodes. Whether it's a morning yoga session or a few minutes of deep breathing, these small acts of self-care can make a big difference.

You'll screw up from time to time by eating something you know you shouldn't have, skipping your fibre or meds, or getting dehydrated. And for that screwup, you may well pay what is hopefully only a small price. And you'll learn from it. It's a reminder that diverticulosis is in your colon for as long as your colon is inside you.

Avoidance tactics are your best defense against known triggers. Planning meals with safe ingredients sets your gut up for success. Don't buy food you know you can't tolerate, even if it tastes great. If you do purchase food you shouldn't eat, as soon as you realize you have done so, give it to a neighbour or a local food bank. Don't let that stuff sit in your house just waiting for a weak moment.

If you are the type of person capable of creating a meal plan, consider that a rare strength. Build a plan that includes foods you know your gut loves and stick to it as much as possible. My ability to create a meal plan consists of nothing more than the typical caveman thinking: "Hunger: Eat." And sometimes the seafood diet: See Food. Eat it. But perhaps you can do better than me.

You don't need to overhaul your life overnight; instead, make slow changes to minimize flare-ups. Incorporate new foods gradually, allowing your gut time to adjust. Similarly, gradually increase physical activity levels to support digestive health. Whether it's a daily walk or a weekend hike, these activities can help keep your gut happy, and the rest of you healthy too. Remember that moderate reasonable exercise is a key part of health care.

Integrating regular health check-ups

Imagine walking into a doctor's office where they greet you like an old friend, not just another chart in the stack. That's the beauty of having a strong relationship with your healthcare provider. Despite the invasion of politicians and corporations, it remains possible to have a small team—or at least one caring clinician—who knows you. A caring doctor-patient relationship transforms doctor visits from distasteful to delightful.

If you have diverticulosis and have had one or more episodes of diverticulitis, well, you've got a chronic disease. Keep in mind that diverticulosis is so common in people—especially over age 50—that it is the normal situation in Western countries. But it is still unwelcome because of the risk of diverticulitis. Getting old is also the normal, but not welcome either. Although getting older beats the only currently available alternative.

If you have a chronic disease, it's time to make sure you have a caring primary care physician (PCP) in America or General Practitioner (GP) in the UK, or whatever your primary care doc is called in your country. If you have a PCP already, one that you like, super. If he or she is not well-versed in your condition, they will become so rapidly.

A good doctor can help you in many ways. He or she knows what screening tests to do and will advise you to avoid bullshit screening tests such as executive physicals, whole body MRIs, and other unnecessary crap that companies market nowadays. She can recommend specialty care when needed and help prevent specialist physicians from over-treating; your PCP can nip that stuff in the bud. Most importantly, your PCP can be efficient because she already knows you. She can help you maintain your health, at least by nagging you to lose weight or eat better, a nag backed by professional credibility. A PCP is one of the few people who can help you overcome some denial you may have about yourself. Almost no one else will tell you that you are a fatty. But your PCP will. He or she might say "You're overweight." Or even "You're obese." Who else is going to tell you the truth about such a thing?

Over time, your PCP will learn who you are and then have rapid insight into what may be going on with you when your health care fails and you seek medical care. That leads to efficiency.

But finding the right PCP is like dating—you might have to swipe left a few times before finding your match. For older folks such as us, *swiping left* is lingo for rejecting a potential romantic partner on a dating app on your cell phone. Love in the age of technology. Anyhow, look for a clinician who has time for you and who listens before they talk. It's okay if the doctor interrupts a bit while you are telling them your story, but only to guide you, not to rush you. Doctors need to get information from you that you may not expect. But they should be asking and *listening* and not preaching or jumping to conclusions.

After you've found your PCP, together you can decide when and how to bring specialists into the mix. Specialists may include a gastroenterologist to deal with chronic constipation concerns or recurrent diverticulitis, radiologists to perform testing, and surgeons to help decide whether to take a section of your colon out. If one has an episode of acute diverticulitis, you have a reasonable chance of having a second and subsequent attacks. One must decide at what point to consider surgery and while some studies suggest that this should not be done until there are more than six attacks, it comes down to a sensible discussion with your doctors - what is right for you given your medical history and risk tolerance. With some effort and diligence, most people can avoid needing the surgeon.

Traveling with Confidence

Traveling can be a joy, a long car ride, a flight to somewhere on your bucket list, or my personal favourite: a sailing vacation. But when your gut has a mind of its own, travel can be a nightmare. The key is preparation, just as you pack clothes and check your passport, have a checklist for your digestive system. Start by packing smart. Bring along whichever medication or foods you use to keep your bowels regular, such as PEG for me, maybe fibre for you. And bring enough for your entire trip and some to spare in case of a delayed return.

Hydration is critical, we cannot state this often enough. On an aircraft, as noted before, one tends to get dehydrated because of the relatively low cabin pressure, dry air and failure to drink enough, so avoid alcohol. If you are going to be on a long trip, take breaks for a stroll. Stop the car every couple of hours, take a long saunter around the airport or train station and pace the aisles. Avoid carbonated beverages before or during the trip, because that gas must find a way out. And yes, when nature calls, answer it, even if it means using the dreaded public restroom. Your gut will thank you for braving the unknown porcelain thrones of the world.

> The flight attendants who provide those tiny bottles of water to you often walk down the aisle farting as they go. They call this "crop dusting." Whenever they crop dust, take it as a reminder to ask them for another one of their tiny bottles of water.

Pack travel-friendly snacks that are kind to your digestive system. Think nuts, seeds, or a fibre- snack like oats. These snacks are not only gut-friendly but also keep you satiated on long journeys.

Choosing the right seat on your flight can make all the difference. Aisle seats are prime real estate for those with unpredictable guts—easy access to the restroom without the awkward shuffle past your seatmates.

We go into this in our chapter on medical and surgical treatment and include some thoughts in Appendix IV, but it is worth mentioning it now also. Nothing says "prepared traveler" like knowing where the nearest hospital is or researching the locations of doctors and pharmacies at your destination before you leave home. And don't forget to brush up on your language skills—knowing how to say "diverticulitis" in the local tongue might just come in handy!

7

The Hunger Pains

Diet & Lifestyle for Diverticulosis to Help Prevent Diverticulitis.

In this chapter, we're diving more into the world of diet and nutrition, focusing on how to keep your stool loose and your digestive system functioning best when you have diverticulosis. The purpose is to either avoid developing or slow down any worsening of diverticulosis and prevent episodes of diverticulitis.

Assure that you poop easily every day and never need to strain: keeping stool loose

Straining to have a stool raises the pressure inside your colon, causing the diverticula to balloon out and can push bits of stool into them, which can cause or worsen diverticulosis and inflame one or more diverticula into diverticulitis. Straining to have a bowel movement is exactly what you *do not want to be doing* if you have diverticulosis. Actually, you do not want to be doing it *ever!* Avoiding the destructive need to *push* requires a constant process of advance planning, 24-48 hours ahead. What you eat and drink two days ago will affect the effort needed to poop today.

Remember that the colon's primary job is to remove water from the stool. If you have diverticulosis, the trick is to interfere with the colon doing its primary job too well. The longer that stool is in the colon, the more time the colon can dry out the stool. The drier the stool, the harder it is. The harder it is, the harder it is to poop it out, meaning the harder you must strain to get the harder poop to hardly move. Hard poop is bad poop.

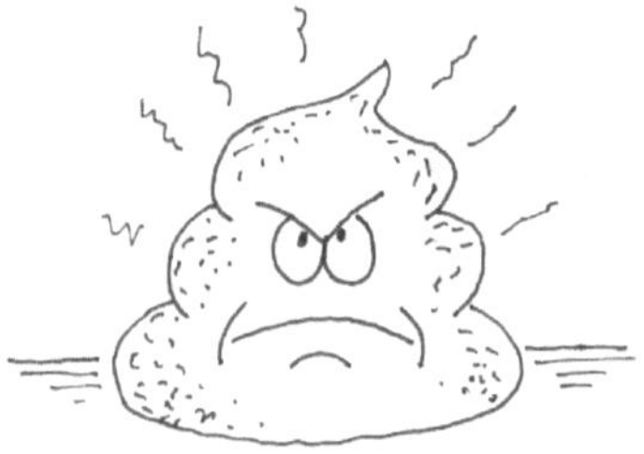

HARD POOP IS BAD POOP

Keeping water in the stool keeps it soft and is important when you have diverticulosis. Keeping stool hydrated is accomplished by 1) keeping yourself well hydrated by ingesting more water, 2) helping the stool to keep its water by ingesting fibre or polyethylene glycol, 3) keeping the colon moving.

For hydration, aim for at least eight glasses of water a day. More on hot days or days when you are exerting yourself.

Water helps a lot, but it helps better alongside dietary fibre.

Most people do well ingesting fibre—material that humans can't digest so it stays in your colon and tends to help improve either constipation or diarrhoea.

Not all fibres are created equal though; soluble fibre, as its name suggests, dissolves in water, forming a gel-like substance that helps keep stool softer. Insoluble fibre adds bulk to the stool and can help firm up stool that is too loose. For people with diverticulosis, soluble fibre is usually the good stuff, but some insoluble fibre is also fine, if you always take it with lots of water.

Fibre not only helps keep diverticulosis calm, but it also has several other benefits; it decreases the creation of hemorrhoids and may lower the risk of colon cancer. It also lowers blood cholesterol by lessening cholesterol absorption. So together with helping ward off diverticulosis it is a miracle food!

You can ingest fibre by either eating fibre-rich foods while drinking lots of water or taking fibre supplements such as psyllium, while drinking lots of water. Water, another miracle food!

It's wise to increase fibre intake slowly, over many weeks. Cranking it up too fast may cause cramping, diarrhoea and general discomfort. Most people can adjust to having more fibre in their diet if they add it slowly enough.

But even starting slowly, some people's guts don't tolerate fibre well because it keeps making them gassy or otherwise uncomfortable. It probably has something to do with the different types of bacteria found in our intestines: we do not all have the same critters lurking there. But it also may have something to do with the type of fibre people eat; some types of gut bacteria digest some fibre and make gas.

If you are one of those folks who do not tolerate fibre well despite starting slowly, there are a couple of options. First, you can consider taking daily polyethylene glycol that we discussed in Chapter 6 instead of the extra fibre, because it does the same thing as soluble fibre when taken with water, but bacteria cannot generally digest it and make gas. Polyethylene glycol has no taste. When it is dissolved in water, it looks just like water. Drinking it is like drinking a mildly thicker version of water. Initially it might feel strange in your mouth, and you might not enjoy it. But you will likely adjust after a week or two. I've been drinking a glass of it every day for years, and I enjoy it. Even if you tolerate fibre perfectly, polyethylene glycol can be very helpful to you.

No, it isn't "natural." But nature sometimes leaves you with diverticulosis and gives you constipation.

The other option is to try a low FODMAP diet; FODMAP stands for Fermentable Oligosaccharides, Disaccharides, Monosaccharides, and Polyols. Now you know why we call it FODMAP. This diet involves removing a whole bunch of FODMAP-containing foods from your diet, then reintroducing one at a time to see if you can identify the guilty party from this line-up. In Appendix II we have briefly set out the FODMAP diet for your convenience.

There are also some foods that tend to prevent constipation that you should consider weaving into your diet:

- High-fibre fruits like prunes, figs, ripe bananas and fresh berries provide natural fibre and water content that promote regular bowel movements. Prunes are particularly effective as they contain both fibre and natural compounds called sorbitol and *dihydrophenylisatin* that have a mild laxative effect. It is also found in prune juice.
- Leafy green vegetables such as spinach, kale, and collard greens are rich in both fibre and magnesium. Magnesium can naturally stimulate bowel movements.
- Legumes including beans, lentils, and chickpeas are good sources of fibre, both soluble and insoluble.
- Whole grains like oatmeal, quinoa, and brown rice contain significant amounts of fibre and nutrients.
- Ground flaxseeds and chia seeds are particularly effective at preventing constipation due to their high mucilage content, which, when mixed with water, helps move stool through the digestive tract.
- Fresh pears and apples, especially with their skins on, provide both soluble and insoluble fibre that aids in maintaining

regular bowel movements. The natural sugars in these fruits can also have a mild laxative effect.

- Kiwi fruit has been shown in studies to be particularly effective at preventing constipation due to its unique combination of fibre, enzymes, and natural compounds.
- Hot beverages, particularly coffee and certain herbal teas like peppermint or ginger tea, can stimulate muscle contractions in the digestive tract and help prevent constipation. Because caffeine can also lead to loss of water via the kidneys, it is smart to drink extra water along with coffee and tea.

Constipating foods

Several types of foods can slow down digestion and lead to constipation. Processed grains like white bread, white rice, and pasta contain less fibre than their whole grain counterparts and can contribute to sluggish digestion. Dairy products, particularly cheese, milk, and ice cream, can be binding for many people, especially those who are lactose sensitive.

Foods high in fat such as fried foods, fast food, and rich desserts can slow down digestion since they take longer to process. Red meat, when eaten in large quantities, can also contribute to constipation because of its high fat and iron content and lack of fibre.

Other foods that commonly cause constipation include unripe bananas and milk chocolate. Additionally, foods with little to no fibre content like chips, crackers, and other highly processed snacks can contribute to the problem. Foods high in salt can lead to dehydration, which is a common cause of constipation. This includes many processed and packaged foods, cured meats, and salty snacks.

It's worth noting that what causes constipation can vary from person to person, and portion size and insufficient water intake play a significant role. Everyone is different. For example, grapefruit is generally considered to help with constipation because it is high in fibre and water content. However, for me personally, there is no more powerful a constipating agent than grapefruit. People are different.

Here is a list of some other stuff you might ingest that may (or may not) cause you constipation.

1. Calcium, found in some antacids like *Tums*, is a well-known constipator. This is why combining it with magnesium (which speeds the gut along) is wise. Some versions of this common antacid contain it. Examples that have both calcium and magnesium in the US and UK are Rolaids, Maalox, Mylanta, Rennies and their generic equivalents.

2. Gluten can cause all sorts of gut problems if you are gluten sensitive (if you have an immune sensitivity to gluten). A doctor can help you figure that out.

3. Sour persimmons (Asian persimmons) contain lots of constipating tannins

4. Underripe breadfruit

5. Alcohol is constipating by causing dehydration and it is also a toxin for the gut.

6. Iron supplements or food containing high amounts of iron (like red meat).

7. Ginseng and Dong quai in large quantities. This is why you need to tell your doctor if you take herbal or alternative medicines

8. Raw chestnuts and acorns.

9. Casava when incompletely cooked

10. Some yams, when incompletely cooked.

Hydrating Foods

Foods that are loaded with water help minimize constipation. And they have another advantage that is relevant to many of us: they are fantastic for weight loss in people who like to eat, like me. The more water, the lower the caloric density of the food. Win win.

1. Watermelon contains about 92% water content. It's rich in electrolytes including potassium and magnesium, which helps keep the stool moving.

2. Cucumber is another excellent hydrating food, composed of approximately 95% water.

3. Citrus fruits like oranges, grapefruit, and tangerines are not only water-rich (about 87-89% water) but also provide essential vitamins and electrolytes. But I can't eat the damn grapefruit for some reason.

4. Lettuce, particularly iceberg and romaine, are composed of more than 95% water. They can contribute significantly to your daily fluid intake.

5. Strawberries and other berries contain around 90% water, along with fibre and antioxidants.

6. Celery is about 95% water and contains natural sodium and potassium, making it particularly effective for hydration. Its fibre content also helps your body retain that water more effectively. I hate celery.

7. Plain yogurt and cottage cheese surprisingly contain about 85-89% water content.

8. Zucchini and other summer squashes are approximately 94% water and can be easily incorporated into many dishes, both raw and cooked.

9. Bell peppers, particularly the sweeter varieties, contain about 92% water. Yum.

Exercise

There are about a gazillion reasons to exercise. Whether it's a brisk walk around the block or a yoga session, movement stimulates gut peristalsis, the process that moves food through your intestines. Exercise not only helps with digestion but also reduces stress, which is a notorious troublemaker in the world of gut health. You don't need to hear more, but I hope you find a way to pull off doing some exercise.

Aim for at least 30 minutes of moderate exercise most days of the week, whether it's walking, yoga, or a combination of both. Consistency is key, so find activities that you enjoy and make them a regular part of your life. And don't forget to listen to your body—if something doesn't feel right, take a break and try again another day.

I don't listen to my own preaching when it comes to exercise. But my lazy nature should serve only as an example of what not to do. Find some way to exercise that you enjoy that feels productive to you. Listen to podcasts while you exercise. Or perform physical labor to attain your exercise. I cut, split and move firewood to use for heating our house in the winter. And I get excellent exercise moving from chair to chair as I sit on my ass.

Finally, listen to your gut—literally. Your body knows when it needs to go. Don't ignore the call to nature. When you feel the urge, don't put it off. Holding it in only gives the colon more time to suck water out of the stool. It makes things harder, in more ways than one.

Stool Softening Checklist: Keeping It Loose and Easy

- **Stay Hydrated**: Drink at least eight glasses of water daily.
- **Eat Fibre-Rich Foods**: Include mostly soluble fibre, or psyllium, or polyethylene glycol.

- **Incorporate Movement**: Engage in regular physical activities like walking or yoga.
- **Avoid Straining**: Listen to your body's natural signals for bowel movements.
- **Monitor Your Diet**: Identify foods that may cause constipation and adjust accordingly.

Some people advocate incorporating foods like yogurt, kimchi, and sauerkraut into your diet as a delicious way to foster a healthy microbiome. These foods are packed with live microbes that, as the good bacteria squeezes through your stomach acid, promote gut health. However, while for *me,* no hot-dog is complete without a generous helping of sauerkraut, the resultant gas makes me regret it and claim I will never do that again. Yoghurt I enjoy, but kimchi? It ain't my cup of tea. And talking of microbes, while antibiotics have saved a gazillion lives, please do not take them if you don't need them; it's not good for your microbiome and increases antibiotic resistance, which is a real problem for the world.

By following these tips, you'll find that keeping your stool loose is an achievable reality. Your bathroom visits will be uneventful, just as they should be. And your diverticulosis is more likely to remain nothing but an occasional bother.

8

The Fast and the Fibrous

Everybody Poops

If you have never read *Everyone Poops* by Taro Gumi, I heartily recommend it. While intended for children I think it is a masterful short tome for adults to peruse too. How parents deal with the transition to self-toileting can impact the child's entire life. Scolding the child for having an accident or rushing defaecation may cause health consequences in adult life.

Have you ever met someone who would not use a toilet at work, in a bar, restaurant, theatre or even a friend's home? Instead of evacuating poop when it sends the message that it needs to come out (the gastrocolic reflex explained in Chapter 1) the person hangs on until they are in a safe space such as their home. During that time, the poop is drying out, getting harder and more difficult to eventually dump. And of course, this raises the pressure inside the bowel, increasing the likelihood of diverticulosis developing.

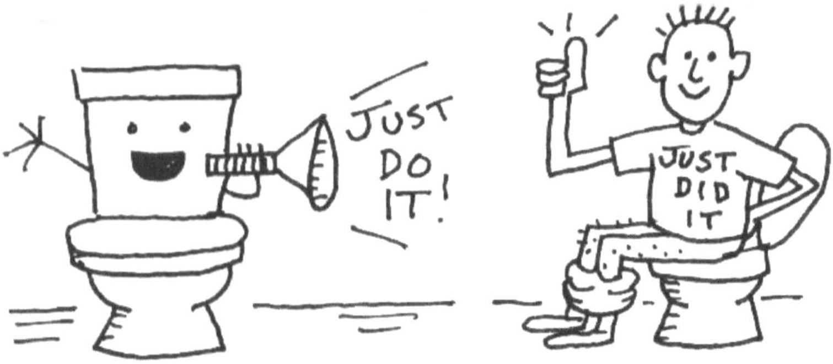

Institutional toilets (schools, offices etc.) very often do little to help people who are embarrassed about going to the loo with gaps under doors, and between cubicles. And nowadays with the move to "gender neutral" facilities I would bet more women are hesitant to enter. A note of caution: I was in an airport once, totally engrossed on a mobile telephone business call as I was walking to my gate and had the urge to deal with my "other business." I saw the toilet sign but was not paying attention and, well, you guessed, walked into the ladies WC. I made a very rapid 180 the moment I saw my error, but was there long enough to note how much more fragrant it was than the usual men's toilets and how taken aback the women occupants were. On another occasion at a trendy restaurant with a unisex toilet, I saw a metal sink running the full length of the room with a constant waterfall effect and a row of cubicles opposite. I popped in, did what I had to do and exited. And there in front of me was a chap quite happily peeing in the sink. Well, he ceased to be happy when two young women entered and, realizing his error mid-stream, he hastily repackaged his equipment and ran out of there like a rat out of a trap. Political correctness comes at a cost it seems.

I have never understood why Americans call the toilet a *bathroom* as we never bathe there. Nor is it a restroom, although that is more germane to this mighty book. As a doctor, if I am a guest in someone's home and ask to use the toilet and find reading material next to the porcelain throne, I can predict bowel problems are likely in the future. You see, if you have time to read a book, browse through a magazine or even check your phone, you are not eating enough fibre or drinking enough water, and thereby assuring that your poop is hard and difficult to evacuate, and so you are going to have to spend time pushing as if you are trying to have a baby. And remember, pushing equals pressure and that is not a good thing! Unless of course you are just sitting there, chilling out and waiting for the magic to happen. The key thing is *do not strain!*

The concept for the flushing toilet was first proposed by Sir John Harington, a godson of Queen Elizabeth 1st in the 16th century. In 1775 Alexander Cumming, a Scot, was granted a patent for a flushing loo and developed the “S” bend that created a water seal, thereby preventing sewer gas from making its way into the room. And around one hundred years later, a London plumber and inventor, Thomas Crapper developed what we would recognize as modern toilets. Although the word “crap” predates Crapper’s life, it was American servicemen based in the UK during World War II who saw the ubiquitous devices branded “Crapper,” christened the trip as “going to the crapper” and shortened the term to the crap itself. Crapper’s shortened name has been used for such diverse concepts as *taking a crap, giving a crap*, and exclaiming *what the crap*.

Why is this all relevant? Well, it isn’t relevant to diverticulosis, but I love history, and it takes me nicely to the delicate subject of hygiene. Having emptied your bowels, close the lid before flushing. Why? Because otherwise that crapper aerosolizes germs, particularly those pressure powered loos that, when flushed, sound like a tornado flipping a freight train.

Flushing an open lid toilet releases a fecal germ plume onto your clothes, the air you breathe, your phone, everywhere. And if your phone accompanies you to the toilet and you then head back to your table at a restaurant, well those germs are going straight into your mouth and that of your companions.

Would you take some action to avoid diarrhoeal disease by 40%, communicable illness by 80% and substantially reduce colds, flus and pneumonia? Wash your hands. Those who hand wash have 24% less respiratory sick days and 51% fewer GI problems. Every hour we touch about 1.5 million germs. And once on your hands they grow like germs!

Ever seen someone leave a restroom without washing their hands? On average, 75% of women and 50% of men wash hands after using the toilet; 20% of people don't wash routinely and 30% don't use soap. Damp hands are *one thousand* times more likely to disseminate bacteria, yet only 20% of those who wash bother to dry their hands. Pressing elevator buttons, handling a banknote or credit card machine, you are effectively touching somebody else's poop. For that matter, when you smell someone's fart, you are breathing into your mouth and nose the molecular effluent that just came out of someone else's butt.

So, while I have your attention talking about diverticulosis, please wash hands regularly for 20 seconds with soapy hot water and dry thoroughly, at the very least after using bathrooms, before and after meals and after physical contact with sick people or items recently touched by sick people.

> I also love Shakespeare. Bill nailed it in *Timon of Athens*: *"Would thou wert clean enough to spit upon" or in modern terms: "you are so dirty I would not have my spit dirtied by touching you!"*

So, the take home messages?

- When you feel the urge to go, go.
- Faeces should come out easily with minimal effort. If it doesn't, drink more and eat more fibre. If you do not, trouble will brew.
- Deep breathing can be helpful as it helps relax the abdominal muscles, reducing the pressure on your colon. Inhale slowly through your nose, letting your belly expand like a balloon, then exhale gently through your mouth. This isn't just about oxygen; it's about signaling to your body that you're in no hurry. Rather like yoga for your gut, minus the incense, elevator music and stretchy pants.
- Changing position can help. In different cultures people poop differently, maybe squatting over the toilet with their bottom well below their knees. It might help to rest your feet on a small stool....so that the big stool can find its way out!
- Being patient can help; in our fast-paced world instant gratification is the norm, but your bowels didn't get that memo. Rushing the process only adds to the pressure, both figuratively and literally. Instead, embrace the art of waiting. Allow your body to take its time, releasing when it's ready, not when you think it should. If nothing's happening, don't panic. Stand up, stretch a little, and try again later.
- If you are really having problems, drink a large warm herbal tea, use laxatives, a glycerin suppository or even a small enema that you can buy over the counter to help the movement.

So, listen to your body and embrace what messages are being sent; dispense with those old bathroom books and commode comics by following our advice. After all, your colon will thank you.

9

When the Gut Hits the Fan

Flare-Ups and Acute Symptoms

The first time you develop a flare-up with acute symptoms it can be frightening, or at least worrisome. Indeed, most people learn about their diverticulosis through two methods: a medical scan or screening endoscopy, or by having that first episode of diverticulitis. That first episode is something you won't have experienced before. It may make you fear you have cancer. It's wise to see your doctor.

If such episodes become a feature of your life you will learn to recognize the characteristics. Once diagnosed with diverticulosis make sure you have a digital or old-fashioned thermometer at home, and if unwell certainly check your temperature. Normal range is typically 36.1-37.2°C (97-99°F), with individual variation. With a glass thermometer, shake it to ensure the column of mercury has moved into the bowl and then insert the thermometer's probe under your tongue, close your lips over it tightly to hold it in place and wait for 5 minutes (unless you have just had a hot or cold drink, in which case use your armpit) or follow the electronic thermometer directions. Also record your pulse rate at the base of the thumb on the wrist by counting how many beats occur in 15 seconds, multiply by four and record both measurements to later inform your doctor.

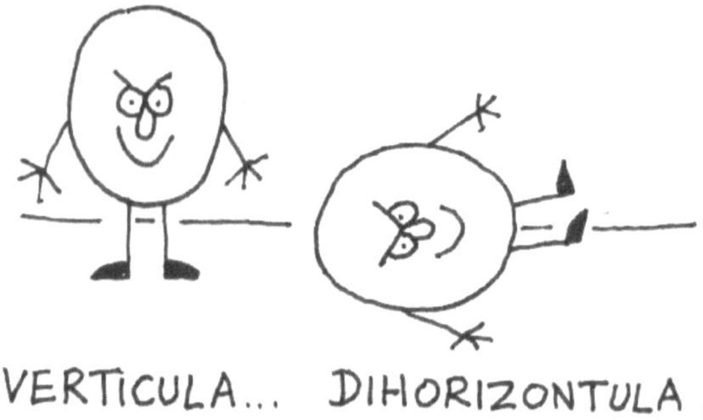

If your temperature is high, pulse rate higher than your normal (for example clicking along at 90 beats per minute or more), pain is severe, you are nauseated or vomiting, and importantly, feel unwell, get thee to a doctor immediately. If medical advice suggests you can stay at home, a heat pack is soothing as it can help relax muscles and reduce pain and tension. And to that end, deep breathing exercises also help as we discussed in Chapter 6: breathe in through your nose, hold for a couple of seconds, then exhale slowly through your mouth. This sends a gentle "all-clear" signal to your nervous system, reducing stress and helping to manage pain.

We discussed high-residue (fibre-rich) and low-residue diets previously in Chapters 5 & 6. If you have an acute episode of diverticulitis, that is the time to follow the low-residue routine to allow the colon to rest. You can check out the sort of foods to eat in Appendix II, but remember, a low-residue diet is the opposite of what you'd normally follow with diverticulosis. It's important to note that this isn't a long-term solution, as a low-residue diet lacks essential nutrients. Drinking fluids is always good as we have stressed repeatedly, and clear broths and herbal teas are a good option. Certainly, avoid caffeine and alcohol, as they can irritate your digestive system and exacerbate symptoms; this is not a bear you want to poke!

Rest and relaxation are your allies during a flare-up: taking short naps can help conserve energy, allowing your body to focus on healing rather than fighting through fatigue. Engaging in light activities, such as reading a book or listening to music, provide a welcome distraction from the discomfort. Keep notes of your symptoms, pulse and temperature and if anything starts to deteriorate, don't hesitate. Get medical attention.

10

Gone with the Gut

Medical and Surgical Treatment

Knowing when to seek medical attention is crucial. If you experience a high fever or severe abdominal pain that refuses to relent, maybe associated with nausea and vomiting, loss of appetite and feeling ill, it is time to call in the cavalry. Symptoms that persist despite your best home remedies may indicate a more serious issue that requires professional evaluation. Remember, it's better to err on the side of caution than to let a flare-up escalate into something more serious. Your health is a priority, and seeking help when needed is a sign of strength, not weakness.

So, let's assume you have made it to the hospital, done the laborious paperwork and fallen into the hands of an expert, what comes next? Well, as you have seen in earlier chapters, the first thing is that they will obtain a history of your condition – do not be irritated if more than one person asks the same question;

this is about ensuring completeness and consistency. People, especially when ill, forget things that can be important. You will then be examined, blood and imaging tests ordered, and intravenous fluids commenced. They may tell you not to eat or drink anything just in case an intervention is called for, because a full stomach poses a risk of aspirating and developing pneumonia under general anaesthesia.

If signposts point to a diagnosis of diverticulitis, intravenous antibiotics as well as pain relievers may be prescribed: the former is more likely if there are signs of generalized infection or your medical status demands it, such as if you are on medications to suppress the immune system or have cancer, diabetes or a chronic inflammatory condition like rheumatoid arthritis. However, over recent years the use of antibiotics has diminished as further data come to light about their relative benefits and risks. You are wise to ask the doctor whether you should have them. If the decision is made, it is typical to use *broad spectrum* antibiotics that target a wide range of bacteria, refining the choice based on further information as it becomes available from blood cultures (where the laboratory endeavours to isolate bacteria that may be growing in your blood) and clinical response. Typically, a 7 – 10-day course of first choice drugs are deployed - trimethoprim/sulfamethoxazole, ciprofloxacin, metronidazole, amoxicillin/clavulanate (Augmentin).

For pain relief, the hospital may start with something simple. But again, be involved in your care and if you are in discomfort, the medication type and dosage can be adjusted.

Abscess

If the clinical pointers lead to a diagnosis of an *abscess* (one or more swollen diverticula that contain pus made up of mucus, bacteria and white blood cells), the decision may be taken to drain the infection. An old expression, to *let out the laudable pus* used to suggest that a wound was healthy if it drained pus, but we know that to not be true. Although it is true that a draining wound is better than a wound filled with pus that is stuck inside an abscess, there is nothing laudable about either.

Once an abscess is well-established, its wall thickens and blood (and antibiotics in the bloodstream) cannot get into the tissue. It is hard to conceive that antibiotics will be able to defeat the process. At this point a decision will be made to drain the infected material. This is usually first attempted by a *percutaneous* technique under the guidance of either an ultrasound probe or within a CAT scanner. The patient may receive some sedation, a suitable area of skin on the abdomen is cleaned, and local anaesthetic injected. Then, a fine needle is inserted by an *Interventional Radiologist*—a doctor trained in using various types of imaging to guide when and how to conduct procedures. Once the needle penetrates the abscess, a wire is placed through the barrel of the needle which is then removed and over this wire the doctor slides a hollow *catheter* to allow the pus to exit. This is held in place on the skin and attached to a drainage bag. If this technique fails, or if the infected area is too large, a surgical approach may be required.

Bleeding

As explained in Chapter 3, an inflamed diverticula can erode into an adjacent artery and cause significant sudden bleeding through the anus. If this is the presenting symptom, the patient may require a blood transfusion and then investigations to identify the leaking artery. Many cases of such bleeding stop spontaneously, but should bleeding continue, the location can be identified on occasion and even treated with colonoscopy. Alternatively, injecting red blood cells tagged with a radioactive isotope can be used to scan for the bleeding site. But nowadays, in sophisticated medical centres, *angiography* is carried out whereby contrast material is injected into the blood while the patient lies in a CAT scanner, which delineates the exact bleeding spot in the gut. At this point, our friendly Interventional Radiologist can guide a catheter to the bleeding spot and inject little pieces of material to block the vessel. In some cases, surgery is required.

Fistula

In Chapter 3 (Complications), we talked about this situation where the inflamed colon can stick to adjacent organs and burrow into them. As one might imagine, faeces leaking into the bladder would cause problems for the entire urinary tract. It can lead to serious systemic infection called *septicaemia*. After acute treatment with antibiotics and fluid resuscitation, surgery will be required.

Stricture

Repeated episodes of diverticulitis from which the patient recovers can lead to scarred bowel that becomes progressively narrower, impeding the passage of poop on its journey to the sewer. This will present as progressively worsening episodes of colicky abdominal pain, loss of appetite, nausea and vomiting, distended abdomen and constipation. On occasion, a skilled operator can stretch up the narrowed section with a balloon under guidance of a colonoscope, but often a surgeon is required to deal with this.

Surgery

Operating on patients with diverticular disease requires an experienced and specially trained doctor, familiar with the various presentations and surgical techniques available. If an operation is performed *electively* (i.e. in a planned manner or non-emergently), there will be time to inform the patient in great detail as to what to expect from surgery, as well as for the patient and physician to consider the alternatives, risks and benefits. Until recent times, it was normal to order bowel preparation, similar to that used before colonoscopy to render the bowel "clean" prior to surgery, but many feel doing this before an operation is unnecessary.

A decision to submit to a planned operation may arise because of repeated episodes of pain, bleeding, fever, or in the setting of the complications listed above.

Of course, in emergency situations such preparation is not an option, but there should still be time to discuss what might transpire during and after surgery, with special focus on whether a *stoma* might be required. The word means "mouth" and refers to the action whereby a part of the bowel is brought to the surface of the skin via an opening in the abdominal wall allowing bowel contents to drain into a bag attached to your skin, diverting faeces from its usual journey outlined in the first chapter of this book. If it is the colon that is so diverted, we call the opening a *colostomy* and if the small bowel, an *ileostomy*. The stoma can either be just one piece of intestinal "pipe" or it can be a *loop* stoma where the opening is an incomplete circumference of the bowel. These stomas are often made as a temporary construct to allow serious problems downstream to settle, after which the plumbing can be returned to normal several weeks or months later. However, on occasion a stoma is permanent, either because of the nature or extent of the disease or because the patient is not fit enough to undergo another operation.

Broadly speaking, the phases of an operation are:

i. General anaesthesia, which includes inducing sleep and complete muscle paralysis so the abdomen can be entered and intubation to allow ventilation to take over as the muscles required for breathing are having a nap.

ii. The skin of the abdomen is cleaned with antiseptic fluid and sterile drapes separate the operative area.

iii. The abdomen is entered.

iv. Diagnosis and extent of diverticulosis, diverticulitis and damage to nearby organs is confirmed and a general look around everywhere else is carried out;

v. The area of diseased colon to be removed is defined based on how much of the bowel is affected, the ability to have two ends to bring together that look and feel healthy and, of course, patient history.

vi. Bring bowel ends together and join them with sutures, staples or other methodology. This joining is called an *anastomosis* and needs to be fashioned cleanly, with no obvious gaps, with bowel that has healthy bleeding edges and is under no tension (see Figure 6).

    i. If the surgeon feels that the anastomosis is at risk of compromise, the disease burden is too high or the patient is quite unwell, they may choose to "protect" the join by making a stoma upstream so that no faeces can pass through the joined bowel until the bowel is reconnected at some later date.

    ii. The most common area for diverticulosis is the sigmoid colon. Sometimes when we operate and find really nasty diverticulitis it is not considered judicious to take care of everything at that time. So, instead of removing the diseased bowel and joining everything together, we isolate the bad part by bringing the bowel to the surface as an "end" colostomy and put drainage tubes into the abdomen so the bad stuff can find its way out. We can then return to fight another day and take care of removing the affected part at that time. Sometimes we can remove the diseased segment but not do a "join" so we bring out the colon as a stoma "upstream" and close off the downstream part of the bowel, usually the top of the rectum. This operation, called *Hartmann's Procedure* after the doctor who developed it, can be a lifesaver.

In recent years *laparoscopy* or "minimally invasive surgery" has been used to access the abdomen. This is where instead of making a large incision, the abdomen is inflated with carbon dioxide such that one looks 9 months pregnant. Small tubes are then placed via tiny incisions at various locations, and through one, a telescope with a video camera attached is inserted, displaying an image of the inside of the belly on screens in the operating room. Then other instruments are placed and any operation as described can be carried out. This approach leads to faster post-operative recovery periods, smaller scars and fewer complications. Laparoscopic operations tend to be more feasible for planned operations when the gut is quiet, because acutely inflamed tissues during an attack can be tricky to deal with laparoscopically, but it is always worth discussing.

Another innovation that has benefitted surgery is the development of a robotic platform that is controlled by the surgeon sitting at a console in the operating area while doing a laparoscopic operation. He or she views the procedure via a 3D screen and can precisely manipulate the instruments with more exactitude than when using direct touch. Again, this is more germane to planned, rather than emergency operations.

Living with a stoma

This possibility will have been discussed before surgery and should appear on the consent form a patient should read and sign before surgery. If a planned operation, there should be time to meet with a *Stoma Therapist,* a specialized healthcare practitioner who can show you what will be involved, mark on your skin the likely location of the opening such that it will not impede a belt line or be uncomfortable. Modern appliances are very effective at minimizing the impact of a stoma, but the most important thing is knowledge—to understand how diet will impact the stoma and how to best protect the skin. And as we cover below, having the right mental attitude will help you live with this inconvenience. I am always moved to quote the famous scientist, JBS Haldane, who not only diagnosed his own bowel cancer, but wrote a witty poem about it called *Cancer's a Funny Thing* in 1964 with the aim of raising awareness of the disease. Given he ended up with a colostomy on his abdomen, the poem includes the lines "So now am I like two-faced Janus, the only god who sees his anus." Finding humour in adversity is a mark of great courage!

Postoperative recovery

Nowadays hospital stays tend to be as brief as possible and much is up to you. Getting mobile early limits the chance to develop complications like chest infections or venous thrombosis and will also get your bowels working sooner. Following doctors' and nurses' instructions and advice is important, but so is ask-

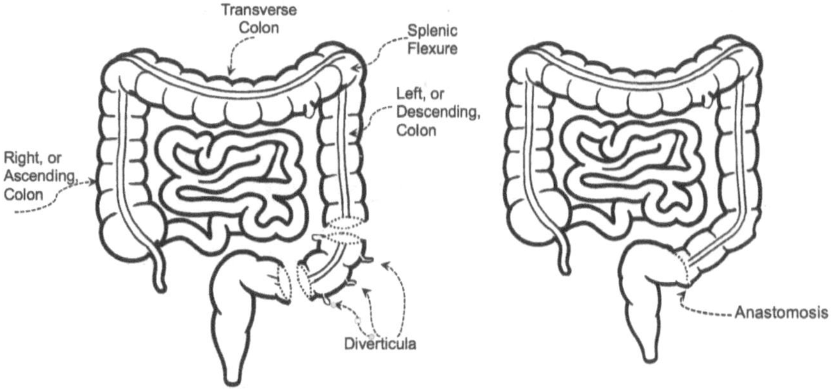

Figure 6. Resection and anastomosis of bowel with diverticula

ing questions and taking care of your mental health. Your colon may have been acting up, but with the right intervention, you'll be back to enjoying life without the constant background noise of digestive distress.

As for post-operative diet, that will depend to some degree on what operation was performed. If the entire colon is removed (rarely required for diverticulosis) and the bowel drains into an ileostomy bag, keeping your faeces soft will not be the issue, it will be the opposite because the colon won't be there to remove water from the stool. If just one section is removed, most commonly the sigmoid, then the stool is likely to be more liquid than before the surgery as there is simply less colon available to absorb water. However, there will likely be some remaining diverticulosis, because we only remove that which must come out. So, it will be wise to stick to a high-fibre diet, lots of fluids and all the other steps that have been recommended to avoid the problem in the first place.

Emotional and Mental Health Support

Dealing with a chronic condition like diverticulosis is a challenge at the best of times, full of "what if?" and "why me?" And now of course you have had to undergo a major operation which can cause its own dis-ease. Think about it: you have pain, have consumed anaesthetic drugs, antibiotics, and analgesics, and are stuck in a depressing hospital away from your loved ones and your routines. All of this can negatively impact mood. And if you are the recipient of a stoma, even if temporary, that will also doubtless play some havoc on your state of happiness.

Recognizing these uninvited emotions is the first step in managing them. Persistent sadness or irritability may start to creep into your daily life. If you find yourself snapping at the toaster for burning your toast or feeling blue on a sunny day, these could be signs that anxiety or depression is making itself at home.

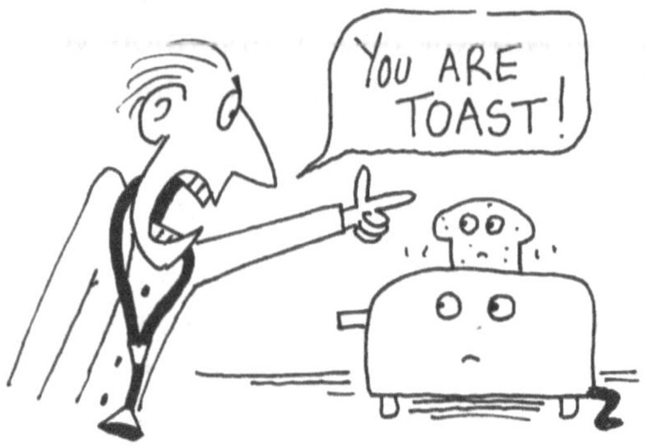

Excessive worry about health or the future can also be a red flag. It's one thing to be concerned about your next doctor's appointment, but it's another to lie awake at night imagining every possible scenario where your condition takes a turn for the worse. If your mind feels like it's stuck on a loop of worst-case scenarios, it might be time to hit pause and seek help. Loss of interest in activities you once enjoyed is another telltale sign. If the idea of streaming your favorite show feels as appealing as watching paint dry, or if you'd rather nap than attend a social gathering you had always enjoyed in the past, it may be time to reassess what's happening upstairs.

Acknowledging these symptoms isn't easy, but it's crucial. It's like finally admitting you need glasses after squinting at road signs for years. Once you recognize the signs, seeking help becomes the logical next step. Engaging with support groups can offer shared experiences and a sense of camaraderie. You're not alone in this, and sometimes hearing someone else's story helps. And for goodness' sake, please let your doctors know. Do not wait until you feel desperate before seeking help.

Reaching out for support is not a sign of weakness; it's an act of courage. Your mental health is a crucial part of your overall well-being, and nurturing it is as important as managing your physical symptoms.

Interactive Element: Mindful Reflection Exercise

1. **Identify Your Emotions:** List any emotions you've been experiencing lately. Are they persistent, or do they come and go?
2. **Spot the Triggers:** Note any situations, thoughts, or events that seem to trigger these emotions. Is there a pattern?
3. **Evaluate Your Support System:** Reflect on who you can reach out to for support. Do you have friends or family to talk to, or might support groups or medical professionals be beneficial?
4. **Set a Goal:** Write down one small step you can take to improve your mental health this week. It could be reaching out to a friend, scheduling a therapy session, or practicing mindfulness. Daily affirmations and journalling have been shown to help; merely repeating phrases like "I am capable" or "I am resilient" or "I am getting better" can foster a more optimistic mindset.

By acknowledging your feelings and taking proactive steps, you can regain control over your mental health, all important steps in your recovery.

We have now covered what might happen if diverticulosis gets out of control and requires the very best that modern medicine can offer to make you better. As we turn the page to the next chapter, we'll explore alternative and complementary therapies.

11

The Sound of Mucus

Healing Through Alternative Therapies

You've heard the phrase, "trust your gut," but when your gut is sick, maybe it's time to not trust it! The question is who and what you can trust in this age of lies, more lies, and damn lies. Do you trust "modern medicine"—also known as allopathy as practiced by Doctors of Medicine? We three doctors freely admit that conventional medicine is a mess. This is not because we don't mean well; it's just that the *business* of medicine, massive costs and shortage of resources get in our way. Do you trust Dr. Google, which is, we doctors shout, a *more* horrible mess? Or do you trust "Alternative" medicine? Well, let's start with what alternative medicine is.

Alternative medicine can be broadly considered as *unproven medicine*. But that then leads to the question, "what does it mean that something is *proven* in medicine?"

And that is a surprisingly difficult question to answer, because, quite truly, not as much is proven in the modern medicine realm as we all like to pretend.

Let's start with what constitutes proof in modern medicine. The allopathic realm has adopted *evidence-based medicine* (EBM). The top tier, gold standard, of proof in the EBM hierarchy is the prospective, randomised double-blind placebo-controlled study. In this type of study, an intervention, such as a medication that researchers hope will be helpful, is tested in a group of patients with a given medical condition or disease, but in a particular way. Some patients are given *placebo*, something that looks like the real treatment but is not believed to influence the body, and some are given the test medication. Neither the doctors nor the patients are supposed to know who is given what. The researchers must, *in advance*, choose outcome variables to measure. The study and the measurements go on that way until complete, and then the results are analysed to see if the test medication did anything compared to the placebo, both in affecting the disease being treated or causing side effects.

There are multiple ways to do this analysis, but the most common is to look at average outcomes of the subjects in the test drug group compared to the placebo group. Let's say we have an imaginary test drug, *Shrinkaglute* which is supposed to make butt size smaller. The study team looks to see if the butt size shrinks more, on average, in the test group than in the placebo group. And they likely examine how many troublesome side effects the test group has compared to the placebo group. If the research design is good enough, and the results positive, this sort of study is taken by doctors and regulatory agencies as the best proof of the efficacy of a therapy.

But there is a big but, whether or not you have a big butt. This type of study mostly looks at the *average* outcome of the group. The big but is that YOU were not enrolled in this study, and you will not have the same biology as the average person enrolled in the study. Your butt may be smaller or bigger than the average person's butt and may respond very differently to this medication than the average person's butt does.

The buttshell of this is that evidence-based medicine is a collectivist construct; it prioritizes and pays heed to group outcomes rather than individual outcomes. This conflicts with the way that medicine should be practiced, in my mind at least. Medicine should be a highly individualized process, because you are a highly individual person. A physician who practices solely evidence-based medicine, which focuses on the outcomes of groups, must ignore much of the variability between people. In fairness, in certain areas of medicine we are moving more to personalized approaches, such as in cancer treatments. The problem is the cost of effectively doing research studies to find out exactly which very expensive drug is best for each individual patient.

Evidence based medicine studies can prove that a drug works for the average person but can't prove that it works for you. What the prospective, randomized, double-blinded, placebo-controlled study may be able to tell us is whether a new therapy *might have a reasonable chance* of doing any good for you as an individual patient.

To determine if a given study is even relevant to you, you need to look at a few factors.

Does the average person in the study bear some reasonable similarities to you as a person, including the same age range, same sex, and the same version of whatever disease it is that you have and want treated? The disease version is very important: for instance, "breast cancer" is not one disease but a range of different types of cancers each of which has many subtypes that impact how to best treat it. There is no doubt that pharmaceutical development has helped us improve or save the lives of countless people, and companies rely on evidence-based medicine to determine if a drug is worth taking to market. The double-blind placebo-controlled study is the best tool available for this purpose, but these studies are in no way perfectly predictive of a medication's usefulness in you.

Another example: there are many types of asthma. If you have one type of asthma and the study is looking at a drug in a totally different type of asthma, then the study is likely irrelevant to you, meaning it cannot tell you anything about the chance that the drug might work for you. But the drug may be approved by regulators like FDA and therefore promoted by the makers as being suitable for treating asthma without being more specific.

Evidence based medicine is not the complete answer for what is proven and what is unproven. But when conducted well, it helps get us in the right direction.

Now that we have characterized conventional medicine, what about the alternative? There are many alternative medicine fields. Homeopathy, Chinese traditional medicine, functional medicine, naturopathy, ayurvedic, acupuncture, and the list goes on. Each has good and bad features. What most, but not all, practitioners of these fields tend to share is a general lack of data proving that their diagnostics or therapies are likely to do any good for you. Many are happy to take your money in exchange for their approaches, although of course there are many well-meaning folks out there. The problem is that practitioners of most alternative fields do not consider it important to undertake the effort of proving that their stuff works. They either don't respect the scientific process, or are in a rush to make money based on hunches and guesses.

Sometimes this is okay. The "let's see if this works in you" method of proving a drug's efficacy in an individual patient has some merits, if the likely benefit outweighs the risk. A particularly big merit is that it is testing the drug IN YOU, as opposed to someone else. Indeed, allopaths (such as MDs in America) often use this method. But the allopath decides to try a drug or therapeutic compound in you based on their knowledge of you as an individual and, whenever possible, informed by how the therapy performed in groups of people similar to you in earlier prospective double-blind placebo-controlled studies scientific studies, and also informed by their clinical experience. In contrast, the alternative practitioner makes the decision based on their knowledge of you, but doesn't have trustworthy scientific data on how other people like you have fared on the therapeutic compound.

Instead of relying on information collected using the scientific method, many alternative practitioners practice *anecdotal medicine*. This is when a clinician has had one patient (or maybe a series of patients) who does well on a given medication or supplement and then assumes that this patients' seeming success means that the therapy is likely to work in you. This differs from the evidence-based methodology in critical ways: 1) there is a very real placebo effect that, if ignored, will make patients and anecdotal medicine clinicians think that a drug has a benefit, even though it does not; 2) the patients whom the alternative clinician has tried the drug on *who do poorly* are unlikely to return for a follow up visit; the clinician therefore doesn't hear about the failures and can easily allow themselves to be misled, and then misleads the next patients either willingly or in ignorance.

There are other alternative practitioners who practice *hypothetical medicine*. As an example, this is where the clinician studies up on some enzyme pathways in the body and the chemicals involved in those pathways and then prescribes nutritional supplements either to try to encourage those pathways to do more or to discourage those pathways from causing harm. The problem with this is enormous, both scientifically and in society. Scientifically, just because some scientist or clinician hypothesizes that an enzyme pathway is relevant to your disease or condition doesn't mean that it is. Rarely do hypothetical medicine practitioners study whether dosing up on a bunch of supplements even affects the enzyme pathway at all. Even more rarely do they try to assess the actual effect on your disease.

Hypothetical medicine is what underlies almost all the supplement industry. Basically, it is a bunch of hypotheses with no testing of these hypotheses by any scientific means. Anyone can make up a hypothesis. *Sucking on sunflower seeds makes people's butts smaller.* There, I just made up a hypothesis. You can make up a hypothesis too. But would you want your doctor doing that and selling you expensive medical interventions based on their potentially lame thinking?

What underlies the massive growth in the supplement field? It is not proof of efficacy, that's for sure! To us, it seems that people are fed up trying to access an impersonal, administratively top heavy and expensive medical system. Some are now rebelling against the authoritarian tendencies of the public health practitioners that became evident during the peak Covid fear period. Further, although there are many good people working in the pharmaceutical industry, any time there is a scandal, trust is eroded, and the purveyors of supplements turn that loss of trust in the system to their profit.

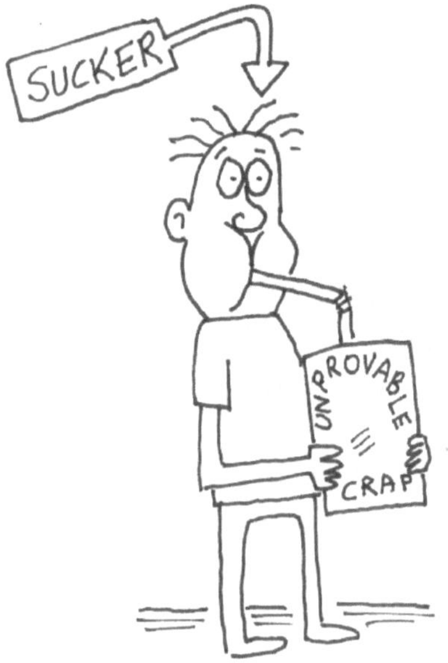

A good rule to apply is that if a clinician or company does not offer any evidence that an intervention can or should work other than anecdotes and patient testimonials, then the intervention is not worth paying for. In ancient times, physicians were only paid if the patient recovered. In Rome if the outcome was not good, *lex talionis,* the law of retaliation, could even be imposed and the unfortunate practitioner could even be put to death. Now I am not suggesting we should go the way of Rome, but it is important that the health of patients is what motivates us, that ethics are the foundation of what we do, and anyone who sells a treatment that cannot be proven to work, and particularly if they don't even care enough to *try* to prove it works, is likely not being ethical.

Those who sell unproven medical interventions prey on people's ignorance, exhaustion, or desperation. Unproven interventions should be cheap, free, or the patient should be paid as a research subject for participating in an experiment. What people shouldn't do is swallow or inject or inhale unproven stuff in an experiment which isn't even a real experiment and pay for the "privilege" of doing so. And yet that is precisely what people are doing when they hand over their cash to buy supplements. By the way, if people stopped buying unproven crap, then the profit motive of the alternative practitioners would encourage them to prove the best of the unproven stuff that are most likely to work. We all would win. But when people pay for placebo, and practitioners profit from placebo, the profit comes best to those who induce the most confidence.

Speaking of confidence, the best purveyors of the unproven are in many ways con artists. They maximize the placebo effect by making patients believe that the stuff works. Then they get those patients to speak loudly and broadly about how well it worked for them, and then other people buy the stuff. So those it "works" in then are recruited to talk the stuff up to help sell it to others, thereby expanding the con. Those in whom the therapy doesn't seem to work aren't invited to say anything. This part of anecdotal and hypothetical medicine is entirely marketing, and fraudulent marketing at that. Whenever you see people saying how wonderfully well some drug or supplement or intervention helped them, you can count on one thing and one thing only: that you are being subjected to intentional manipulation, that they are trying to turn you into a sucker.

It's not a sign of health consciousness to be taking a bunch of unproven supplements. It might be a sign of being a bit of a sucker. And one thing is for sure, these supplements can be very costly and mostly just make your urine expensive and the seller wealthy.

All that being said, some supplements have some proof behind them, like medications, and indeed may work as well as big pharma drugs, or better. But those supplements have been subjected to some sort of testing.

Perhaps the best way to sort out whether a drug or supplement works or not in a person is, when possible, to do a double-blind placebo-controlled test *on that person*. For example, the patient takes one pill a day for a month, either the active drug or placebo, and researchers measure the outcome. Then change to the other pill, which looks the same, take that for a month and measure the outcome. Do that a couple of times and it is possible to gain reasonable knowledge about the drug's effect on this one person, mostly unclouded by the placebo effect. It's not perfect, but if done carefully with good placebo that appears and tastes just like the active drug, you have perhaps the best proof of efficacy in the individual patient who are we wanting to treat. But this technique only works when the intervention (drug or supplement) has actions that can be measured in a month or so. If it takes years to see benefit or side effects, this won't work.

So, what do we know about alternative treatments for diverticulosis and diverticulitis? Not a lot. Because we three doctors, despite our critical approach to everything until shown to work, have some disdain for those who never even try to prove their stuff works.

Probiotics and Prebiotics

Although there have been a couple of dozen studies on probiotics in diverticulosis and diverticulitis, the studies haven't proven much of anything. The studies haven't entirely disproven the potential use either. But this lack of ability to prove the stuff is helpful means, at least, that the stuff they have tested isn't very helpful. There may be some modest benefits or modest harms.

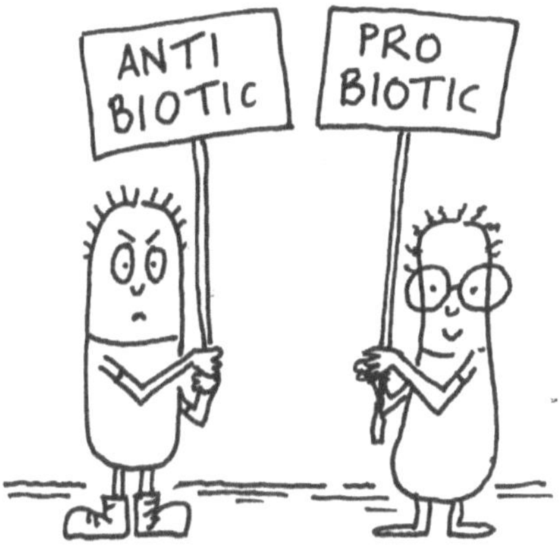

Probiotics are live bacteria and yeasts that play the role of friendly neighborhood microbes. Prebiotics, on the other hand, are the indigestible fibres that feed these beneficial bacteria. Together, they can, theoretically, create an environment that helps digestion and nutrient absorption, lessen risk of overgrowth by bad bacteria, and maybe even decrease unhelpful inflammation. Probiotics may help with medication absorption and vitamin production, while prebiotics improve calcium absorption and may help to keep gut lining healthier.

> Supplements often have on their label some phrase allowed by regulators such as "support immune function" or "support healthy gut." These phrases pretty much mean nothing at all. At most they mean that someone hypothesized that they may be useful. Keep in mind that "supporting" immune function may be good for fighting infections but bad for people who have a disease that results from inflammation such as rheumatoid arthritis or allergic asthma. Basically, the labeling of supplements is mostly hogwash.

Now, before you start stocking up on probiotic and prebiotic supplements, let's talk about how to choose them so that as you experiment you can try to compare apples to apples. One issue is whether the probiotic is formulated in a way that the bacteria can survive the harsh acid environment of the stomach. To give you a perspective, think of your stomach like a pool in one of the James Bond movies, a villain falls in, thrashes about, screams ......and disappears. That is your stomach. If the probiotic bacteria all get killed in the stomach, then there is not a lot of value to be had. Essentially, they are just no more than foods, sources of calories. But there are some good bacteria like *acidophillus* that, as their name implies, tolerate the harsh stomach environment: (acid + *philo* - love), and can make it through. Yogurt usually contains this bacterium.

There is a Probiotic Checklist available that is relatively useless that goes something like this, with our comments in italics.:

- **CFU Count**: Aim for a product with a high CFU (Colony Forming Units) count, a measure of how many bacteria is present. *Although unproven to be of use, the suggestion here is that if the stuff works, more of the stuff might be better than less. Possibly. Probably. But maybe not. One of the known side effects of pre-biotics and probiotics is that they could make you gassy, which is bad for diverticulosis. So, watch out for that!*

- **Strain Specificity**: Choose strains known for your specific digestive needs. *There is some knowledge of this, but we don't know much. How do we know your specific digestive needs? How can we choose the right strain? We are doctors but certainly not experts in you or which bacteria your personal gut needs.*

  - **Lactobacillus acidophilus (L. acidophilus)**: *Maybe lessens antibiotic-induced diarrhoea and helps with digestive tract infections.*

  - **Saccharomyces boulardii (S. boulardii)**: *May help prevent diarrhoea and bacterial ulcers.*

  - **Bifidobacterium (B. lactis)**: *May be useful to lessen constipation and irritable bowel syndrome.*

- **Label Check**: Look for quality assurance certifications on the label. *Who knows? Such assurances could well be bogus.*
- **Expiration Date**: Ensure supplements are fresh and potent. *Not that an expiration date assures either of these.*
- **Dietary Compatibility**: Consider any dietary restrictions or allergies. *This one is pretty obvious. If the stuff makes you worse, or makes you sick, don't take it.*

Summary: Try probiotics and pre-biotics if you want. Be as objective as you can. Try not to mislead yourself about how much they help or hurt you. Please don't tell others how well it works for you, because doing so is scientifically useless and serves as free marketing for those who make money without going to the effort to prove their stuff works.

Herbal Remedies and Natural Supplements

In the realm of anecdotal medicine, these remedies are like the ancient myths: filled with tales of the miraculous. Take chamomile, for instance. People often brew the dainty flower into tea, declaring it the peacekeeper of the digestive system, though scientific backing for this is elusive. Then there's ginger, the spicy root that's claimed to tackle nausea and indigestion. There are many such foods and herbs that appear to have effects on the gut, which makes some sense.

The historical foods we eat have gone through thousands of years, even tens of thousands of years of non-scientific anecdotal testing. Someone in the tribe would try some bit of a plant, and if he or she didn't puke or die, and the stuff tasted okay, other members of the tribe might give it a try, and it becomes food. Some foods have appeared to have benefits in treating some illnesses, and through unscientific trial and error, some of those have survived the test of time in the marketplace of ideas. Chinese traditional medicine, although seemingly entirely unscientific with its focus on Qi, has the longest history (5,000 years) of people trying stuff. Over that long period of time, practitioners have figured out that some foods and herbs do seem to help. Ayurvedic medicine likewise seems full of bogosity but has a long history of trial and error which separated some wheat from a lot of chaff.

Homeopathy drives us a bit crazy. Here's why. True homeopathy involves taking supplements that work to mimic the disease process you are having, under the assumption that your body knows best, so help it along. If you have diarrhoea, the homeopath will give you something that would make you have more diarrhoea. Homeopath indeed means "same as the pathology." There may be something to that concept sometimes. But homeopathy has only been around for a bit more than a century. It doesn't have the multiple millennia of trial and error to find what really works. Importantly, they still don't do testing in any scientific way. Then it gets really squirrelly. Because in true homeopathy, the preparers of the substances dilute the substance until there isn't any left. And then they have the nuts to say that diluting it *even further* makes it even stronger. They offer some claptrap about transferring the energy of the supplement to the water molecules. This is utter hogwash. The strongest homeopathic substances are nothing but water.

> The term "homeopathy" has more recently been used by marketing people beyond the meaning of true homeopathy to now include regular supplements, some of which have been proven useful, most not proven one way or the other. Those false homeopathic compounds actually have something in them other than magic water. So maybe they will work better than true homeopathy (which cannot work at all). But the marketing bums never test them, since so many people are paying for the unproven stuff anyway.

Sometimes scientists will study what a long history of trial and error has led us to believe may be useful. When the scientific method is deployed, sometimes it proves that the stuff works. Sometimes it mostly disproves it.

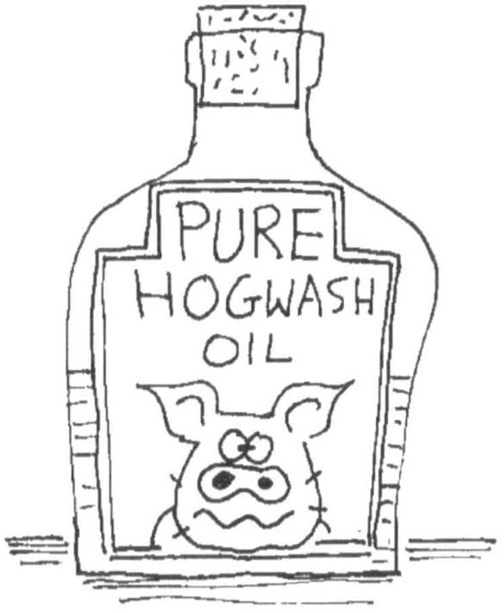

Enter the example of turmeric, the golden spice that's been touted rather aggressively as an anti-inflammatory agent and in the recent past as a means of preventing bowel cancer. Proof is mostly lacking, and there have been some scandals. In the 1980 through 2010's, suppliers in India put dyes that contained lead into turmeric to enhance its vibrant colour. It caused abdominal pain, vomiting, kidney and brain damage and even death. Oops. More recently, studies that purported to show turmeric as helpful in fighting cancer were retracted when further scrutiny exposed the research to be flawed. However, by that time many companies were marketing curcumin—the "active" ingredient in turmeric—as an anti-cancer medication, supported only by wildly inaccurate claims. This tells us that although science can help to prove stuff works, it can also be used to confuse or mislead whether due to fraud or poor science.

Scientists who can profit off their work may have some extra motivation to fake data and behave in an unethical or criminal manner. But such abuses are rare, and for every one of these egregious actors there are many hard-working men and women with curious minds and good moral compasses who publish around 3.5 million scientific articles every year, increasing our scientific knowledge dramatically and spending gazillions of money in the process. Yes, science is not the end-all-and-be-all, but it is a damn sight better than snake oil salesmen touting unproven or even dangerous "cures." The best course of action is to enjoy turmeric as a food and don't pay for it as a medicine.

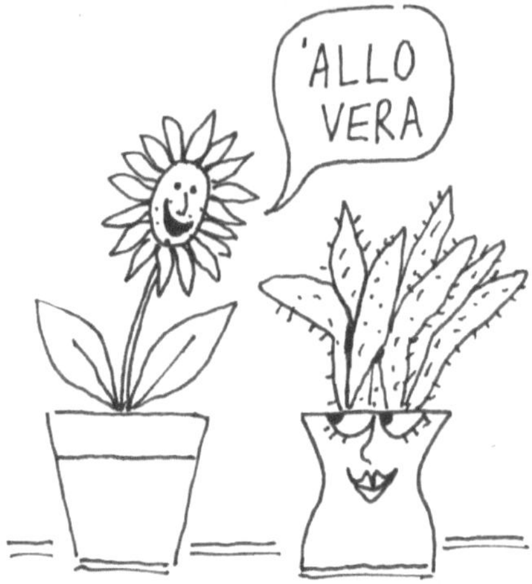

Aloe vera, often hailed as a natural anti-inflammatory, is another contender in the supplement arena. Most folks are familiar with its use as a topical gel for sunburns, but aloe's potential doesn't stop at the skin. When consumed in juice form, it's said to soothe the digestive tract and reduce inflammation. Note the language, "it's hailed as" and "it's said to soothe." But does it do anything, or do people just hail it and speak about it soothingly? It's hard to say. Aloe vera seems to function as a prebiotic, keeping good bacteria happy in the gut. It also contains a bunch of latex, which serves as a laxative, although beware if you are allergic to latex. There are some safety concerns with long term use. Keeping the gut moving and un-constipated is a good thing to do to decrease diverticulitis flares, although there are better ways than slurping aloe vera to accomplish this. There is some theoretical, but clinically unproven anti-inflammatory activity of aloe vera, but even if that theory holds up, the effect will be small and limited. Overall, aloe vera for diverticulosis/diverticulitis is probably not worth the expense. Also, obviously, don't ingest some aloe preparation that is not designed for swallowing.

Peppermint, with its soothing menthol, is known for its ability to relax the muscles of the gastrointestinal tract. Peppermint can help alleviate symptoms like bloating and gas. There is a reasonable understanding of how menthol acts on various nerves in the body and a very long history of it being tested in non-scientific methods over millennia. So, this one may be worth trying. The use of menthol should be brief—a few days at a time.

Slippery elm, derived from the inner bark of the elm tree, is known for its goopy texture when mixed with water – there is a marvelous $100 word to describe it: *mucilaginous*. This gooey concoction coats the digestive tract, creating a soothing barrier that may help calm irritated tissues. People have used slippery elm for generations to address ailments ranging from sore throats to digestive grumblings, and while science hasn't caught up to Granny's wisdom, many swear by its soothing effects.

Before you let your hypothetical herbalist loose on the supplement aisle, it's wise to consult healthcare providers. These professionals can help ensure that your chosen remedy won't clash with your current medications. While herbs might seem harmless because they sprout from Mother Earth, remember, so do opium, cyanide, arsenic and radon. Supplements can interact with medications in surprising ways. For instance, St. John's Wort, often touted for its mood-boosting properties, can make your birth control pills no longer control birth. (Incidentally, what a strange name, *birth* control? It's really pregnancy control, right? *Oral contraceptives* are the far better name, but I digress). Similarly, some supplements can thin your blood, a concern if you're already taking anticoagulants, or block or augment the effects of anticoagulant drugs. So, before you start your herbal adventure, have a chat with a healthcare professional. They'll help you navigate potential pitfalls and ensure your quest for gut health doesn't end in unforeseen complications.

Herbal treatments offer intriguing possibilities, blending tradition with potential scientific backing. As we transition to the next chapter, we'll explore more about personalized strategies for digestive health—because one size doesn't fit all when it comes to your gut.

Mindfulness and Digestion

Your gut and brain have a complex relationship. They communicate through an intricate gut-brain axis about which we are learning a great deal. Stress, though, can throw a wrench in this dialogue, causing symptoms like bloating and discomfort. By practicing mindfulness, you can turn down the volume on stress and tune in to the whispers of your gut, establishing more peaceful digestion. Studies have shown that mindful practices, including meditation, may even help regulate the bugs living in your gut—the *microbiome*—assisting with food digestion and reducing stress markers like cortisol.

This connection between mind and gut isn't just a one-way street. When you practice mindfulness, you enhance this gut-brain axis. It can be as simple as taking a deep breath, releasing tension and allowing your thoughts to merge seamlessly with your body's signals.

To get started on this journey to internal Zen, consider incorporating mindfulness techniques into your daily routine. One popular method is body scan meditation, where you lie down and mentally travel from head to toe, checking in with each part of your body. As you scan, you may discover tension you didn't even know you had. This practice not only relaxes your mind but also helps you become more attuned to your body's needs. Then there's breath-focused meditation, a technique that uses the breath as an anchor, helping you stay grounded when life feels like a whirlwind. By simply focusing on your inhalations and exhalations, you can create a calm center amidst the chaos.

For beginners, establishing a meditation routine can be daunting. Starting with short, guided sessions of just five to ten minutes can make a world of difference. Apps like Headspace or Calm offer a treasure trove of guided meditations for those new to the practice. I know I have banged on about proof. Well, there is some proof that these digital mentors can help you navigate the ins and outs of meditation without the pressure of achieving enlightenment on your first try and help your health in the process. Aim to meditate at the same time each day, whether it's a morning ritual with your coffee or a wind-down session before bed. By making meditation a regular part of your routine, you may soon notice its transformative effects on both your mind and gut.

Regular mindfulness practice has a cornucopia of psychological benefits. Mindfulness can increase your resilience against stress. It also enhances emotional regulation, helping you respond better to stressful stimuli. By cultivating this emotional and stress awareness, you'll find it easier to navigate both minor irritations and major life changes, while maintaining an inner equilibrium.

Yoga and Movement Therapies

Yoga is an ancient practice that you can use to twist, bend, and breathe your way to digestive harmony. We have already discussed the parasympathetic nervous system in Chapters 6 and 8. You will recall that this system activates when it is time to rest and digest, whereas its opposite number, the sympathetic system tells your gut to butt out as there is some serious fighting or fleeing to attend to. The parasympathetic system relies on acetylcholine, a chemical messenger that tells your gut to relax and your food to move along. Indeed, drugs that block acetylcholine are used to slow down the gut when you have diarrhoea. Yoga taps into this system, promoting relaxation, enhancing circulation, and boosting motility in your gastrointestinal tract by getting the parasympathetic to power up, and the sympathetic to power down.

Bear in mind that yoga was initially all about meditation and mental approaches. Only recently did the mat and stretchy pants come into play! So, the brain part we have already covered, but what about the poses you should deploy? The first recommendation is to seek help from people who care enough about yoga to learn about it a lot. You don't need to be a contortionist to reap the benefits of yoga; you just need a mat and a bit of patience. Supposedly, Cat-Cow Pose is a great place to start. As you move between arching your back like a cat and dipping it like a cow, your spine gets a gentle massage, and your gut receives a nudge to get moving. Another gem is the Seated Forward Bend. Sit tall, reach for your toes, and feel the stretch ease bloating and discomfort.

Tai Chi and Qi Gong offer alternative paths to digestive nirvana. Tai Chi, with its slow, deliberate movements, is like a moving meditation, calming the mind and reducing stress. Tai Chi can even—maybe, perhaps, possibly—enhance your gut flora diversity, which may, perhaps, possibly, promote a healthier digestive environment. Qi Gong, on the other hand, focuses on balancing the flow of Qi, or energy, throughout the body. It's not about rigorous exercise; it's about gentle, flowing movements that align body and mind.

Integrating these practices into your daily routine doesn't require a lifestyle overhaul. Start by setting aside a few minutes each day for some gentle stretching or a quick Tai Chi session. It can be as simple as rolling out your yoga mat in the living room or joining an online class in the comfort of your pyjamas.

If you're new to these practices, consider joining a local class or finding a community online. The camaraderie and guidance can be a great motivator, turning what might feel like a solitary exercise into a shared journey. Remember, it's not about perfection; it's about progress. Over time, you'll find these practices becoming a natural part of your routine, like brushing your teeth or scrolling mindlessly through your phone.

And while we're here, let's not forget the importance of listening to your body. Not every pose or movement will suit everyone, and that's okay. The goal is to find what works for you, what feels good, and what helps your gut find its happy place. So, try different things, experiment, and embrace the journey with a sense of humor and curiosity. And after all, your gut is with you for life.

12

Game of Groans

Common Myths and Misconceptions

You know those urban legends, like the one about the alligator in the sewer or the idea that swallowing gum means it stays in your stomach for seven years? Well, diverticular disease has a few myths of its own, and they're just as persistent, if not as entertaining. Somewhere along the line, these misconceptions have taken root, and like weeds in a garden, they need a little tugging to set things straight. And given the internet is an echo chamber, once you have searched one kooky idea, you can guarantee those magical algorithms will continue to feed you more of the same. So, why don't we dig in.

One of the most stubborn myths is the idea that if you have diverticulosis, it's only a matter of time before you're dealing with diverticulitis. It's like saying having a driver's license means you're destined to crash your car. Sure, diverticulosis involves those little pouches in your colon, but they're not necessarily ticking time bombs. We wrote this book to help people avoid contracting the disease or helping prevent progression.In fact, most people with diverticulosis never experience diverticulitis. According to the Cleveland Clinic, only 10 to 25% of people with diverticulosis develop diverticulitis, and most cases are mild. It's like buying a lottery ticket; you have the pouches, but that doesn't mean you're winning the diverticulitis jackpot anytime soon. A study from the Veterans Affairs Greater Los Angeles Healthcare System found that only 4.3% of patients with diverticulosis developed diverticulitis over an 11-year period.

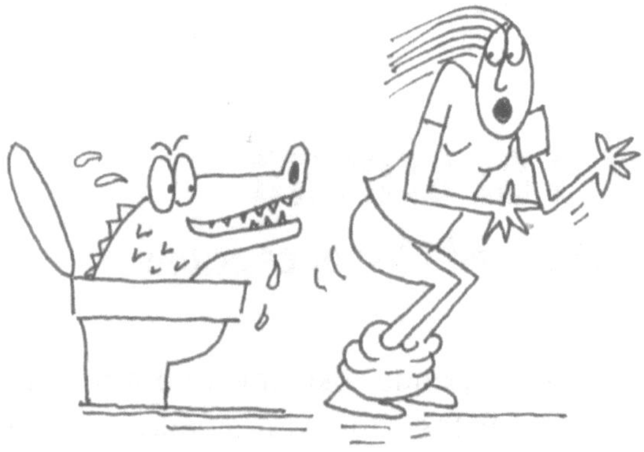

This myth likely stems from a combination of fear and a lack of understanding the relationship between the two conditions. The truth is diverticulosis is often totally silent and symptom-free, or the effects are so mild people discount them. Of course, it merits being taken seriously and treated with respect, meaning a high-fibre diet and regular check-ups. Frankly those are sensible things to do anyway.

In the USA, diverticulitis accounts for around 150,000 hospital admissions per year and in Britain, around 50,000, so it carries a substantial burden. Younger patients might be at a slightly higher risk, but the odds still favor a peaceful coexistence with those pesky pouches.

Myth-Busting Checklist: Diverticulosis and Diverticulitis

- **Diverticulosis ≠ Diverticulitis**: Having diverticulosis doesn't mean you'll develop diverticulitis.
- **High-Fibre Diets Do Help**: Eating nuts, seeds, and popcorn is safe and can prevent diverticulitis.
- **Most Cases are Mild**: Only a small percentage of diverticulosis cases result in diverticulitis, and most are manageable without drama.
- **Lifestyle Matters**: Regular exercise and avoiding constipation can reduce your risk.
- **Myth Origins**: Fear of the unknown and outdated information contribute to misconceptions.

We mentioned nuts and seeds in Chapter 6 and how they can be helpful or a pain in the rear end. Somewhere along the line, someone started the rumor that these delightful snacks were the arch-nemesis of diverticulosis. The myth suggests that given a diverticulum is a little opening from the inside of the colon, swallowing something small and hard could lead to it getting stuck in that hole, blocking drainage of mucus and possibly leading to an abscess. A reasonable idea, but as we covered earlier, having a hypothesis is just the start; one must prove whether it's true. And for most people, it isn't true. Nuts and seeds are not only safe, but they are also part of a high-fibre diet that helps prevent diverticulitis.

These myths persist because they've been repeated so often that they start to sound true. It's like the old wives' tale that if you go outside with wet hair, you'll catch a cold. We accept them because they're simple explanations for complex issues. But the reality is, diverticular disease is more nuanced. It requires a balanced approach to diet, lifestyle, and medical care. Ignoring fibre because you fear a seed might take a detour into a diverticulum is like refusing to swim because you might encounter a shark in your local pool.

However, as discussed in Chapter 11, the chance of subsequent attacks of diverticulitis increases with each episode. The truth about diverticulosis and diverticulitis is that they're manageable with the right information and a little common sense. You don't need to live in fear of every almond or sunflower seed. Instead, focus on maintaining a balanced diet rich in fruits, vegetables, and whole grains. And lots of water. And remember, while myths can be persistent, they're no match for the facts. With the right understanding, you can navigate the world of diverticular disease without getting lost in the fog of misinformation.

13

The Latest Poop Scoop

Staying Informed

A doctor may know a lot about disease, but it is the patient who knows the most about his or her body. The doctor-patient relationship therefore should be, as John suggested in Chapter 6, a collaborative and close one where each (the patient and the doctor) has specific responsibilities: the patient to truthfully report symptoms and adhere to treatment; the doctor to listen and, using the best available information, act.

Physicians commit to a lifetime of learning, attending courses and conferences, reading the medical journals and undergoing regular evaluations to ensure they are up to date with latest advances. But the patient can also keep informed because, simply put, it is their body – and we each only get one. If both doctor and patient stay informed about scientific advancements, they keep each other honest and ensure the right diagnostic tests and treatments are instituted. A patient can go too far and drive their doctor bonkers constantly flooding them with ideas that are just not relevant, but it is sensible to be prepared for each appointment with a written list of questions about new concepts one has discovered.

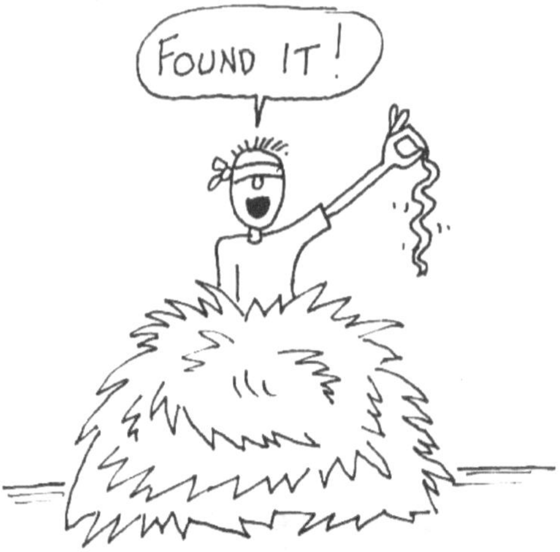

FINDING A NOODLE IN A HAYSTACK.

Transforming your understanding and management of diverticulosis and diverticulitis will also help you understand and adhere to recommended treatment regimes.

Navigating the sea of health information available today is like trying to find a needle in a haystack—while blindfolded. And merely googling can be misleading and worrying. We're not yet sure about how AI will guide patients, but googling is like casting a net of all one's fears and phobias, or all one's denials, and clicking only on those articles that most tickle your fanciful fancies. Yes, you could always go to medical school, train as a gastroenterologist or surgeon and plough through the scientific literature. But given you probably have better things to do and there are over 30,000 reputable medical journals with around 300 focusing on gastroenterology, maybe there are other solutions.

Following respected health organizations and experts on social media can provide a more digestible flow of information, in the USA and online Dr. Sanjay Gupta of CNN or our own podcast at Join the Docs (available on Spotify, Apple Podcasts, social media and at our website, www.jointhedocs.com). Like Sanjay, we are delivering curated information and not selling vitamins, supplements or other similar products. So maybe a good time to get a word from Nigel Guest.

"Hopefully you have found this book to be a helpful and understandable guide to all aspects of diverticular disease. As our eminent surgeon Jonathan said at the beginning, the inspiration for this volume came from our esteemed colleague John selflessly providing a physician's view of his own illness and experience.

As a humble Family Doctor my observation is that while diverticular disease is common, and we see it often, severe diverticulitis and the surgical ramifications are thankfully not. If you already have diverticulosis, the advice regarding managing your condition and preventing deterioration are invaluable. I cannot emphasise enough that if you experience severe abdominal pain and tenderness, feel ill, have a raised temperature and possibly vomiting don't mess about...see a doctor now!

If you are reading this as a non-sufferer, the prevention advice is sound; consume a good diet, loads of fibre, loads of fluids (water ideally), keep your weight down and exercise. Poo daily, checking to ensure your poop is large and fluffy. Don't sit on the loo for hours and strain or you'll be reading our book on haemorrhoids next. Eat tomatoes, seeds and seedy fruit and vegetables with impunity. Be sensible and don't obsess. Enjoy your bowels, look after them and they will look after you. Enjoy life; live long and prosper. I guess that is a vegan thing, similar to Vulcans but without the pointy ears."

Of course, it's not just about passively consuming information. Engaging with patient advocacy groups can provide a dynamic way to stay informed. These groups focus on each given disease and in this case The International Foundation for Gastrointestinal Disorders (https://iffgd.org/) for instance, is a treasure trove of resources. They host webinars and conferences, offering a platform where you can learn directly from experts and fellow patients. Participation in these events not only boosts your knowledge but also connects you with a community that understands your experiences, offering support and camaraderie in what might otherwise feel like a solitary battle.

Online forums and discussion groups also play a pivotal role in this information ecosystem. They're the virtual equivalents of a town hall meeting, everyone can participate, and you can share experiences, ask questions, and learn from others who have been there, done that, and got the t-shirt. Whether it's debating the merits of the latest dietary fad or swapping stories about the best probiotic on the market, these platforms are invaluable. Just remember, like any good dinner conversation, take everything with a grain of salt and verify facts before making health decisions. To quote President Ronald Reagan, "Trust, but verify."

It is worth creating your personal list of go-to research resources including adding trusted health influencers on social media for accessible advice and updates. Include patient advocacy groups such as IFFGD for community support and engagement. Finally, list any forums or online communities you find particularly helpful. Keep this list handy, updating it as you discover new sources. This will be your personalized map, guiding you through.

We hope you have enjoyed:

Some Important Medical Sh*t: Diverticulosis & Diverticulitis

Despite our incompetence with computers, we are aware that you can't click on hyperlinks in a printed book, but we hope you will pop over to: www.jointhedocs.com and wander around our website. There is a lot of cool stuff to discover.

Don't try clicking on that link if you are reading a paperback right now. It will just make your fingertip sore.

You can subscribe to our free podcasts, read anything new we add to the information in this book, as well as easily access hyperlinks from our appendices consisting of super resources that may help you with your condition.

Additionally, you can see what we are planning next, whether that's our next book – because we now have the publishing bug – or a live show, or anything else. You can also drop us a line at info@jointhedocs.com with suggestions for what we should cover, or any other suggestions as long as they are kind and anatomically feasible. We can't promise we will be able to oblige, but if we do, Join the Docs will try to make you laugh while teaching what we know about a plethora of medical shi*t.

Until next time, stay safe, stay well, stay curious!

The Docs.

P.S. Don't forget to read the appendices and the mighty professional glossary that follow.

APPENDIX I

PREPARING FOR YOUR DOCTOR VISIT

What questions might your doctor ask you?

A detailed medical history helps the doctor to better understand your overall health and determine the most appropriate course of action for diagnosis and treatment. It's important to be as thorough and honest as possible when answering these questions to ensure the best care, so reviewing these questions ahead of time best prepares you to answer fully. It's in your best interest!

It's always helpful to take notes during your visit, bring a trusted family member or friend with you, and ask for clarification if something isn't clear. The more information you gather, the better prepared you'll be to manage your condition.

Here are the key elements that a doctor typically asks about during a detailed medical history:

1. Chief Complaint (Reason for Visit)

- What brings you in today?
- When did you first notice the problem or symptoms?
- Have your symptoms changed over time?
- How severe are your symptoms (e.g., mild, moderate, severe)?
- What are you most concerned about regarding your symptoms?

2. History of Present Illness (HPI)

- Can you describe your symptoms in more detail?

- When did the symptoms start, and how have they progressed?
- Are the symptoms constant, or do they come and go?
- What makes your symptoms better or worse (e.g., eating, exercise, rest)?
- Do you have any other symptoms that seem related?
- Have you tried any treatments or medications? If so, did they help?

3. Past Medical History

- Do you have any chronic medical conditions (e.g., diabetes, hypertension, asthma)?
- Have you had any previous hospitalizations, surgeries, or medical procedures?
- Have you experienced any major illnesses or injuries in the past?
- Do you have a history of any gastrointestinal problems, cardiovascular conditions, or other relevant conditions?
- Do you have any ongoing treatments or medications from previous health issues?

4. Family Medical History

- Do any close family members have a history of chronic conditions like heart disease, cancer, diabetes, etc.?
- Has anyone in your family had similar symptoms or conditions?
- Are there any hereditary conditions known to run in your family (e.g., genetic disorders, cancer)?
- What is the health status of your parents, siblings, and children?

5. Medications

- What prescription medications are you currently taking (including dosages and frequency)?
- Are you using any over the counter (OTC) medications, such as pain relievers or antacids?
- Do you take any vitamins, herbal supplements, or other non-prescribed products?
- Have you ever had any allergic reactions to medications?

6. Allergies or Intolerances

- Do you have any known allergies to foods, or environmental factors?
- Have you experienced any allergic reactions in the past?
- Are there any other sensitivities or intolerances you have (e.g., to certain foods or substances)?

7. Social History

- Do you smoke, and if so, how much and for how long?
- Do you drink alcohol? If so, how much and how often?
- Do you use recreational drugs or have a history of substance use?
- What is your occupation, and does it involve any exposure to hazardous substances or stress?
- Are you physically active? What types of exercise do you do and how often?
- What does your diet typically consist of? Are there any dietary restrictions or preferences?
- Do you have any significant lifestyle habits, such as sleep patterns or relaxation techniques?

- Do you live alone, or do you have a support system at home?
- What is your mental and emotional well-being like (e.g., stress, anxiety, depression)?

8. Review of Systems (ROS)

This involves asking about various body systems to identify any symptoms you may have missed or not reported yet. Some areas covered may include:

- **General:** Fever, weight loss, fatigue, night sweats
- **Skin:** Rashes, itching, changes in moles or skin
- **Eyes:** Blurry vision, eye pain, redness, dryness
- **Ears, Nose, Throat:** Hearing issues, sinus problems, sore throat, nasal congestion
- **Cardiovascular:** Chest pain, palpitations, shortness of breath, swelling in legs
- **Respiratory:** Cough, wheezing, difficulty breathing
- **Gastrointestinal:** Abdominal pain, nausea, vomiting, diarrhea, constipation, blood in stools, heartburn
- **Genitourinary:** Painful urination, blood in urine, incontinence, frequency of urination
- **Musculoskeletal:** Joint pain, stiffness, muscle weakness
- **Neurological:** Headaches, dizziness, numbness, tremors, memory issues
- **Psychiatric:** Mood changes, anxiety, depression, sleep disturbances
- **Endocrine:** Excessive thirst, hunger, heat/cold intolerance, sweating

- **Haematologic:** Easy bruising or bleeding, anemia, lymph node swelling

9. Immunizations

- Are your vaccinations up to date (e.g., flu, pneumonia, tetanus, COVID-19)?
- Have you had any recent vaccinations or immunizations?

10. Preventive Care and Screening

- Have you had routine screenings, such as mammograms, colonoscopies, or blood pressure checks?
- Do you follow a regular schedule for preventive care?
- When was your last physical exam, and did it include screening for common diseases?

11. Sexual and Reproductive History (if applicable)

- Are you currently sexually active, and do you use any contraception?
- Do you have any history of sexually transmitted infections (STIs)?
- Do you have any history of pregnancy, complications, or gynecological issues?
- Have you had any issues with your menstrual cycle (if applicable)?

12. Mental Health History

- Do you have any history of mental health disorders, such as depression or anxiety?
- Have you ever received therapy or counseling?
- Are you currently experiencing any mood or behavioral changes?

- Have you had any thoughts of self-harm or harming others?

What questions should you ask your doctor about diverticulosis?

Being diagnosed with diverticulosis can bring up many questions and concerns. And although we have covered them in this book, there is no harm in repetition, so here is a comprehensive checklist of questions to ask your doctor to better understand your condition and make informed decisions about your health. If we've done a good job, you will know most of these answers from a general point of view and be prepared to focus those generalities on the unique person that is you.

Understanding diverticulosis

1. What exactly is diverticulosis, and how did I develop it?
2. What is the difference between diverticulosis and diverticulitis?
3. Is diverticulosis a serious condition?
4. Are there any risk factors or underlying conditions that caused my diverticulosis?
5. How common is diverticulosis, and are there any genetic factors involved?
6. Can diverticulosis progress into diverticulitis or other complications?

Symptoms and Diagnosis

1. What symptoms should I look out for that may indicate a flare-up or complication?
2. Is it common to have diverticulosis without any symptoms?

3. What tests or screenings will be done to monitor my condition?
4. How frequently should I have follow-up appointments or tests (like a colonoscopy)?

Treatment and Management

1. Is there a specific treatment for diverticulosis, or is it mainly about prevention?
2. What dietary changes should I make to manage my condition (e.g., intake, avoiding certain foods)?
3. Should I take any medications to manage symptoms or prevent complications?
4. Are there any over the counter or prescription medications I should avoid?
5. Will I need to make lifestyle changes, such as exercise or weight management?

Diet and Nutrition

1. How much should I be consuming each day?
2. Should I increase or decrease the amount of fruits, vegetables, or grains in my diet?
3. Are there any foods I should avoid completely (e.g., nuts, seeds, popcorn)?
4. Is there a specific diet plan or meal plan I can follow to manage diverticulosis effectively?
5. Can a high-fibre diet help prevent complications or flare-ups?

6. Should I consider a supplement, and if so, which one is best?

Complications and Risk Factors

1. What are the potential complications of diverticulosis, and how can I prevent them?
2. How likely am I to develop diverticulitis or another complication in the future?
3. If I develop diverticulitis, what are the treatment options and potential risks?
4. Are there any signs that would indicate a more serious complication, such as bleeding or infection?

Lifestyle and Daily Life

1. Can I continue my normal activities, including work and exercise, with diverticulosis?
2. How much exercise is recommended to help manage the condition?
3. Can stress or emotional factors affect my condition?
4. Is there any impact on my ability to travel or socialize due to dietary restrictions or symptoms?

Medications and Supplements

1. Are there any medications I should take to prevent symptoms or complications?
2. What role do antibiotics or pain relievers play in managing diverticulosis or diverticulitis?

3. Are there any natural supplements or remedies I should consider, such as probiotics or herbal treatments?
4. How do I safely manage other medications I am taking, particularly if they affect digestion or the gut?

Long-Term Outlook and Prevention

1. What is the long-term outlook for people with diverticulosis?
2. What can I do to lower my risk of complications or flare-ups in the future?
3. How often should I be monitored for possible complications?
4. Is surgery ever required for diverticulosis, and if so, under what circumstances?
5. Are there any signs or symptoms that would indicate I need to contact you right away?

Other Considerations

1. Should I be concerned about any other conditions or diseases (e.g., colorectal cancer, irritable bowel syndrome) in relation to my diverticulosis?
2. What resources, such as support groups or literature, can you recommend for people with diverticulosis?
3. Are there any alternative therapies or treatments that may help with managing diverticulosis?
4. Should I seek a second opinion, or is the treatment plan you've outlined sufficient for my condition?

APPENDIX II

VARIOUS DIETS

(1) HIGH FIBRE DIET TO AVOID DIVERTICULOSIS AND EXACERBATIONS

By regularly consuming these -rich, anti-inflammatory foods, you can help prevent diverticulosis and reduce the risk of diverticulitis flare-ups.

1. **Increase intake gradually** to avoid bloating or gas.
2. **Drink plenty of water** to help move smoothly through the digestive system.
3. **Chew food well** to aid digestion and absorption.
4. **Avoid highly processed and low- foods** (*white bread, processed meats, fried foods, excessive dairy*).
5. **Work out what works for you to have at least one effortless daily bowel motion.**

(i) Whole Grains: *Help maintain regular bowel movements and prevent constipation, reducing pressure in the colon*

- **Oats** (*Steel-cut oats, rolled oats, oatmeal*)
- **Whole Wheat Bread & Pasta** (*100% whole wheat bread, whole wheat pasta*)
- **Brown Rice & Quinoa**
- **Barley & Bulgur**
- **Bran Cereals** (*Wheat bran, oat bran, bran flakes*)

(ii) Legumes: (Beans, Lentils, and Peas) *Excellent sources of and plant-based protein to support gut health*

- **Lentils** (*Brown, green, red, yellow lentils*)
- **Beans** (*Black beans, kidney beans, navy beans, pinto beans, chickpeas, soybeans*)
- **Peas** (*Green peas, split peas, snow peas*)

(iii) Fruits: *Provide vitamins, and antioxidants to reduce inflammation and promote gut health*

- **Apples (with skin)**
- **Pears**
- **Berries** (*Raspberries, blackberries, blueberries, strawberries*)
- **Oranges & Citrus Fruits**
- **Bananas** (When ripe, *rich in prebiotics for gut bacteria health*)
- **Avocados** (*High in and healthy fats*)
- **Prunes & Dried Fruits** (*Eat in moderation to prevent excessive gas*)

(iv) Vegetables: *Promote gut motility and help prevent diverticulosis flare-ups*

- **Leafy Greens** (*Spinach, kale, Swiss chard, arugula, romaine lettuce*)
- **Cruciferous Vegetables** (*Broccoli, Brussels sprouts, cauliflower, cabbage*)
- **Carrots & Sweet Potatoes**

- **Bell Peppers**
- **Zucchini & Squash**
- **Beets**
- **Cucumber (with skin)**

(v) Nuts & Seeds (In Moderation, if Well-Tolerated): *Previously thought to cause diverticulitis, but now recognized as beneficial sources of and healthy fats*

- **Almonds**
- **Walnuts**
- **Chia Seeds**
- **Flaxseeds**
- **Pumpkin Seeds**
- **Sunflower Seeds**

(*Tip:* **Soak chia and flaxseeds before eating** to aid digestion.)

(vi) Healthy Fats: *Help reduce inflammation and promote smooth digestion*

- **Olive Oil (Extra Virgin)**
- **Avocado Oil**
- **Fatty Fish** (*Salmon, mackerel, sardines, tuna*)
- **Nuts & Seeds** (*Almonds, walnuts, flaxseeds, chia seeds, sunflower seeds*)

(vii) Probiotic-Rich & Fermented Foods: *Support a healthy gut microbiome, reducing inflammation and improving digestion*

- **Yogurt (with live cultures)**
- **Kefir**
- **Sauerkraut**
- **Kimchi**
- **Miso**
- **Tempeh**
- **Kombucha**

(viii) Hydrating Foods & Fluids: *Helps work effectively to prevent constipation and diverticulosis complications*

- **Water (At least 8 glasses daily)**
- **Herbal Teas** (*Ginger tea, peppermint tea, chamomile tea*)
- **Coconut Water**
- **Cucumber & Watermelon** (hydrating and rich in fibre, cucumber more so)
- **Soups & Broths** (*Vegetable broth, bone broth*)

(ix) Lean Proteins: *Easy to digest and help maintain gut health without excess fat that can slow digestion*

- **Skinless Chicken & Turkey**
- **Lean Cuts of Beef & Pork** (*Sirloin, tenderloin, pork loin*)
- **Eggs**

- **Fish (Fatty Fish for Omega-3s)** (*Salmon, sardines, tuna*)
- **Tofu & Tempeh** (*Great plant-based protein sources*)

(x) Herbs & Spices with Anti-Inflammatory Properties: *Help soothe digestion and reduce inflammation*

- **Ginger**
- **Turmeric**
- **Garlic**
- **Cinnamon**
- **Oregano**
- **Peppermint (if no GERD symptoms)**

(2) SAMPLE LOW RESIDUE DIET

Breakfast: Start your day with a bowl of plain oatmeal or cream of wheat, topped with a small amount of honey for sweetness. Pair it with a cup of herbal tea to keep things gentle.

Lunch: Enjoy a bowl of chicken broth with some plain crackers on the side. Sip slowly and let the warmth comfort your belly.

Snack: Nibble on a small serving of gelatin or a peeled banana for a touch of sweetness.

Dinner: Opt for baked chicken or fish served with a side of white rice. Add a splash of lemon for flavor without the flare-up.

Hydration: Keep a bottle of water or herbal tea by your side throughout the day, ensuring you stay hydrated without overloading your system.

(3) FODMAP

FODMAP stands for Fermentable Oligosaccharides, Disaccharides, Monosaccharides, and Polyols. These are types of carbohydrates that some people have difficulty digesting. These carbs are notorious for being poorly absorbed in the small intestine, leading to fermentation by gut bacteria, which in turn produces gas bloating, abdominal pain, and irregular bowel movements. For those with diverticula, this can exacerbate symptoms; by adopting a low-FODMAP diet, you can minimize the production of these gases, reducing bloating and discomfort and keeping your digestive system calmer.

We won't go into depth about FODMAP in this book but will provide a summary. If you need to dig into it, there are plenty of online resources and various AI tools are happy to help or at least pretend to be happy.

Because everyone is different, the FODMAP diet is commonly implemented in three phases designed to personalize the diet for you. Figuring out your FODMAP diet is a bit of a pain in the ass, but some pain in the ass now can serve to prevent there being a larger diverticulitis pain in your ass later.

1. Elimination Phase (4 weeks): You remove all high-FODMAP foods from your diet. Common high-FODMAP foods include:
    - Certain fruits (apples, pears, mangoes)
    - Some vegetables (onions, garlic, mushrooms)
    - Dairy products containing lactose
    - Wheat-based products
    - Legumes
    - Sweeteners like honey and high-fructose corn syrup

2. Reintroduction Phase (6 weeks): You slowly and systematically reintroduce FODMAP foods, one category at a time, to identify which ones cause unpleasant symptoms.

3. Personalization Phase: You create a long-term eating plan based on your results, incorporating foods you tolerate well while avoiding or limiting problematic ones.

Low-FODMAP foods that are typically safe include:

- Rice, quinoa, and oats
- Most meats and fish
- Eggs
- Many vegetables like carrots, cucumbers, and potatoes
- Certain fruits like strawberries and oranges
- Lactose-free dairy products

APPENDIX III

MEDICATIONS

1. LAXATIVES

Come in several classes listed below with chemical names first and some sample trade names

(i) Stool Softeners (Emollient Laxatives): *Increase water penetration into stool, making it easier to pass*

- **Docusate Sodium** (*Colace, DulcoEase*)
- **Docusate Calcium** (*Surfak*)
- **Docusate Potassium** (*Dialose*)

(ii) Lubricant Laxatives: *Coat stool to reduce water absorption and ease passage*

- **Mineral Oil** (*Fleet Mineral Oil Enema, Kondremul*)

(iii) Saline Laxatives: *Draw water into the intestine via osmotic action, promoting bowel movement*

- **Magnesium Citrate** (*Citroma, LiquiPrep*)
- **Magnesium Hydroxide** (*Milk of Magnesia*)
- **Magnesium Sulfate** (*Epsom Salt*)
- **Sodium Phosphate** (*Fleet Phospho-Soda, OsmoPrep*)

(iv) Hyperosmotic Laxatives: *Increase water content in the intestines, commonly used for bowel cleansing*

- **Glycerin Suppositories** (*Fleet Glycerin Suppositories*)
- **Polyethylene Glycol with Electrolytes** (*GoLytely, MoviPrep, NuLytely*)
- **Lactulose** (*Enulose, Kristalose, Constulose*)
- **Sorbitol** (*Arlex, Sorbilax*)

(v) Peripherally Acting Mu-Opioid Receptor Antagonists (PAMORAs): *Used to treat opioid-induced constipation by blocking opioid effects on the gut*

- **Methylnaltrexone** (*Relistor*)
- **Naloxegol** (*Movantik*)
- **Naldemedine** (*Symproic*)

(vi) Secretagogues (Chloride Channel Activators & Guanylate Cyclase-C Agonists): *Increase chloride and fluid secretion in the intestines to promote movement*

- **Lubiprostone** (*Amitiza*)
- **Linaclotide** (*Linzess*)
- **Plecanatide** (*Trulance*)

(vii) Serotonin 5-HT4 Receptor Agonists: *Enhance intestinal motility by stimulating serotonin receptors*

- **Prucalopride** (*Motegrity*)
- **Tegaserod** (*Zelnorm*)

2. MEDICINES TO BE CAUTIOUS OF IF YOU HAVE DIVERTICULITIS

List of Medicines That Should Be Taken with Caution in Diverticulosis, categorized by class, with chemical names and common trade names in brackets. Talk to your doctor about what might be relevant to you!

(i) Non-Steroidal Anti-Inflammatory Drugs (NSAIDs): *Increase risk of diverticular bleeding and perforation*

- **Ibuprofen** (*Advil, Motrin*)
- **Naproxen** (*Aleve, Naprosyn*)
- **Aspirin** (*Bayer, Ecotrin*)
- **Diclofenac** (*Voltaren, Cataflam*)
- **Indomethacin** (*Indocin*)
- **Meloxicam** (*Mobic*)

(ii) Opioid Analgesics: *Slow gut motility, increasing risk of constipation and diverticular complications*

- **Oxycodone** (*OxyContin, Roxicodone*)
- **Hydrocodone** (*Vicodin, Norco, Lortab*)
- **Morphine** (*MS Contin, Kadian*)
- **Codeine** (*Tylenol with Codeine*)
- **Fentanyl** (*Duragesic, Sublimaze*)
- **Tramadol** (*Ultram, ConZip*)

(iii) Anticholinergic & Antispasmodic Agents: *Reduce gut motility, leading to constipation and worsening diverticulosis symptoms*

- **Hyoscyamine** (*Levsin, Anaspaz*)

- **Dicyclomine** (*Bentyl*)
- **Atropine/Scopolamine/Hyoscyamine/Phenobarbital** (*Donnatal*)

(iv) Iron Supplements: *Can cause constipation and irritation of the colon*

- **Ferrous Sulfate** (*Feosol, Slow Fe*)
- **Ferrous Gluconate** (*Fergon*)
- **Ferrous Fumarate** (*Ferretts, Hemocyte*)

(v) Calcium Supplements & Calcium-Containing Antacids: *May contribute to constipation, worsening diverticulosis symptoms*

- **Calcium Carbonate** (*Tums, Caltrate, Os-Cal*)
- **Calcium Citrate** (*Citracal*)

(vi) Laxatives: *Stimulant laxatives may irritate the colon; bulk-forming laxatives should be taken with sufficient water to avoid obstruction. Safer alternatives include* ***osmotic laxatives*** *like polyethylene glycol (Miralax) or stool softeners like docusate (Colace))*

- **Bisacodyl** (*Dulcolax, Correctol*)
- **Senna (Sennosides)** (*Senokot, Ex-Lax*)
- **Cascara Sagrada** (*Nature's Way Cascara Sagrada*)

(vii) Corticosteroids: *Long-term use may increase risk of diverticular bleeding and perforation*

- **Prednisone** (*Deltasone, Rayos*)
- **Methylprednisolone** (*Medrol*)
- **Dexamethasone** (*Decadron*)
- **Hydrocortisone** (*Cortef, Solu-Cortef*)

(viii) Proton Pump Inhibitors (PPIs): *May alter gut microbiota, increasing risk of complications*

- **Omeprazole** (*Prilosec*)
- **Lansoprazole** (*Prevacid*)
- **Esomeprazole** (*Nexium*)
- **Pantoprazole** (*Protonix*)
- **Rabeprazole** (*Aciphex*)

(ix) Antidepressants (Certain Types): *Some may slow gut motility, leading to constipation and worsening symptoms*

- **Tricyclic Antidepressants (TCAs)**

    Amitriptyline (*Elavil*)

    Nortriptyline (*Pamelor*)

    Imipramine (*Tofranil*)

- **Selective Serotonin Reuptake Inhibitors (SSRIs)** (*Generally safer but may cause diarrhea in some cases*)

    Paroxetine (*Paxil*) - may cause constipation

    Fluoxetine (*Prozac*) - may cause diarrhea

(x) Antipsychotic Medications: *May cause severe constipation, increasing risk of diverticulitis*

- **Clozapine** (*Clozaril*)
- **Olanzapine** (*Zyprexa*)
- **Quetiapine** (*Seroquel*)

3. MEDICATIONS THAT MIGHT BE USED IN ACUTE DIVERTICULITIS

Summary of Treatment Approach Based on Severity:

Mild Cases – Oral antibiotics (if needed), acetaminophen, hydration, low- diet during flare

Moderate Cases – Oral or IV antibiotics, pain management, possible hospitalization

Severe Cases – Hospitalization with IV fluids, IV antibiotics, possible surgery

(i) Antibiotics: *Used to treat bacterial infection in complicated or moderate-to-severe diverticulitis although mild cases* may not require antibiotics as per newer guidelines

- **Metronidazole** (*Flagyl*) – Effective against anaerobic bacteria
- **Ciprofloxacin** (*Cipro*) – Often combined with metronidazole for broad coverage
- **Levofloxacin** (*Levaquin*) – Alternative to ciprofloxacin
- **Amoxicillin-Clavulanate** (*Augmentin*) – Can be used as monotherapy
- **Trimethoprim-Sulfamethoxazole (TMP-SMX)** (*Bactrim, Septra*) – Alternative in certain cases
- **Piperacillin-Tazobactam** (*Zosyn*) – Used in severe hospital cases
- **Ertapenem** (*Invanz*) – Carbapenem used in complicated infections

(ii) Pain Relievers (Analgesics): *Used to manage pain and discomfort.*

- **Acetaminophen (Paracetamol)** (*Tylenol, Panadol*) – Preferred first-line pain reliever
- **Tramadol** (*Ultram, ConZip*) – For moderate pain when acetaminophen is insufficient
- **Hydrocodone-Acetaminophen** (*Norco, Vicodin*) – Used in more severe pain cases (*use with caution due to constipation risk*)

Avoid: NSAIDs like **Ibuprofen (Advil, Motrin)** and **Naproxen (Aleve)** due to risk of gastrointestinal bleeding and perforation.

(iii) Antispasmodics: *Help relieve cramping and spasms in the colon during acute inflammation*

- **Dicyclomine** (*Bentyl*) – Reduces intestinal spasms
- **Hyoscyamine** (*Levsin, Anaspaz*) – Helps with colonic muscle relaxation

(iv) Stool Softeners & Laxatives (Only in Recovery Phase, Not During Acute Attack): *Avoid and laxatives during an active flare, but stool softeners may be used to prevent straining.* *Avoid:* Stimulant laxatives like **Bisacodyl (Dulcolax)** and **Senna (Senokot)** during acute episodes

- **Docusate Sodium** (*Colace*) – Stool softener to ease passage
- **Polyethylene Glycol (PEG 3350)** (*Miralax*) – Used cautiously post-recovery for stool regulation

(v) Intravenous (IV) Fluids: *Used in hospitalized patients with severe diverticulitis who cannot tolerate oral intake*

- **Normal Saline (0.9% NaCl)** – Maintains hydration
- **Lactated Ringer's Solution** – Restores electrolyte balance

- **Dextrose 5% in Water (D5W)** – Provides energy in prolonged NPO (nothing by mouth) patients

(vi) Anti-Emetics (For Nausea & Vomiting): *Used if nausea is present due to inflammation or antibiotic side effects*

- **Ondansetron** (*Zofran*) – Serotonin antagonist for nausea
- **Metoclopramide** (*Reglan*) – Helps with nausea and gastric motility

(vii) Proton Pump Inhibitors (PPIs) (If Needed for Acid Control): *Used if reflux is present or NSAID drugs are being used, but not directly needed for diverticulitis treatment*

- **Omeprazole** (*Prilosec*)
- **Pantoprazole** (*Protonix*)
- **Esomeprazole** (*Nexium*)

(viii) Surgery-Related Medications (If Severe Complications Occur): *Used in case of abscess formation, perforation, peritonitis, or bowel obstruction requiring surgery*

- **Opioid Pain Relievers** (*Morphine, Hydromorphone (Dilaudid)*) – Used postoperatively
- **General Anesthetics** (*Propofol, Sevoflurane*) – For surgical intervention
- **Thromboembolism Prophylaxis** (*Heparin, Enoxaparin (Lovenox)*) – Prevents blood clots in hospitalized patients

APPENDIX IV

EDUCATION

Your best bet for improving your condition. Here we include suggestions for further reading and support:

United Kingdom (UK) Resources

NHS: Diverticular Disease and Diverticulitis

Comprehensive information on symptoms, causes, diagnosis, and treatment.

Website: https://www.nhs.uk/conditions/diverticular-disease-and-diverticulitis/

Guts UK: Diverticular Disease & Diverticulitis

Information on the condition, management, and dietary advice.

Website: https://gutscharity.org.uk/advice-and-information/conditions/diverticular-disease/

Patient.info: Diverticulosis and Diverticulitis

Overview of the condition, including symptoms and treatments.

Website: https://patient.info/digestive-health/diverticula-diverticulosis-diverticular-disease-diverticulitis

NHS Inform (Scotland): Diverticular Disease and Diverticulitis

Information on symptoms, causes, and treatments.

Website: https://www.nhsinform.scot/illnesses-and-conditions/stomach-liver-and-gastrointestinal-tract/diverticular-disease-and-diverticulitis

Bowel Research UK: Diverticulitis and Diverticular Disease

Research-based insights into symptoms and treatments.

Website: https://bowelresearchuk.org/about-bowels/other-bowel-disorders/diverticulitis-and-diverticular-disease/

University Hospital Southampton NHS: Patient Information on Diverticular Disease

Detailed patient leaflet explaining the condition.

Website: https://www.uhs.nhs.uk/media/UHS-website-2019/Patientinformation/Endoscopy/Diverticular-disease-and-diverticulitis-989-PIL.pdf

West Suffolk NHS: Diet and Diverticular Disease

Advice on dietary management for diverticular disease.

Website: https://www.wsh.nhs.uk/CMS-Documents/Patient-leaflets/NutritionandDieteticService/Diet-and-Diverticular-Disease.pdf

Milton Keynes NHS: Dietary Advice for Diverticular Disease

Advice on how to modify diet to manage symptoms.

Website: https://www.mkuh.nhs.uk/patient-information-leaflet/dietary-advice-for-diverticular-disease

NHS: The Eatwell Guide

General dietary advice beneficial for diverticulosis.

Website: https://www.nhs.uk/live-well/eat-well/the-eatwell-guide/

British Dietetic Association (BDA): Diverticular Disease

Evidence-based dietary guidance for diverticulosis.

Website: https://www.bda.uk.com/resource/diverticular-disease.html

United States (USA) Resources

MedlinePlus: Diverticulosis and Diverticulitis

A government-provided health resource covering symptoms and treatments.

Website: https://medlineplus.gov/diverticulosisanddiverticulitis.html

National Institute of Diabetes and Digestive and Kidney Diseases (NIDDK): Diverticular Disease

Comprehensive information on diagnosis, symptoms, and diet.

Website: https://www.niddk.nih.gov/health-information/digestive-diseases/diverticulosis-diverticulitis

Mayo Clinic: Diverticulitis

Trusted medical advice on causes, symptoms, and treatment.

Website: https://www.mayoclinic.org/diseases-conditions/diverticulitis/symptoms-causes/syc-20371758

Johns Hopkins Medicine: Foods for Diverticulosis and Diverticulitis

Expert dietary recommendations.

Website: https://www.hopkinsmedicine.org/health/wellness-and-prevention/foods-for-diverticulosis-and-diverticulitis

American College of Gastroenterology (ACG): Diverticulosis and Diverticulitis

Gastroenterology expert insights.

Website: https://gi.org/topics/diverticulosis-and-diverticulitis/

UCSF Health: Diverticular Disease and Diet

Guidelines on how to eat with diverticular disease.

Website: https://www.ucsfhealth.org/education/diverticular-disease-and-diet

NIDDK: Eating, Diet, and Nutrition for Diverticular Disease

Government recommendations on nutrition.

Website: https://www.niddk.nih.gov/health-information/digestive-diseases/diverticulosis-diverticulitis/eating-diet-nutrition

UpToDate: Patient Education – Diverticular Disease (Beyond the Basics)

A physician-trusted medical resource.

Website: https://www.uptodate.com/contents/diverticular-disease-beyond-the-basics/print

Cleveland Clinic: Diverticular Disease

Digestive health resource with treatment and prevention strategies.

Website: https://my.clevelandclinic.org/health/diseases/10352-diverticular-disease

Harvard Health Publishing: Diverticulitis Diet

Guidance on what to eat and avoid during a flare-up.

Website: https://www.health.harvard.edu/diseases-and-conditions/diverticulitis-diet

Others

1. **Advocate for Digestive Hea**lth https://iffgd.org/get-involved/advocate-for-digestive health/
2. **Top 10 U.S. Healthcare Influencers to Follow on Social Media** https://www.carecloud.com/continuum/healthcare-influencers-to-follow-on-social-media/
3. **Understanding the Link Between Chronic Disease and mental health** https://www.nimh.nih.gov/health/publications/chronic-illness-mental-health
4. **Recovery & Support for Diverticular Disease** https://nyulangone.org/conditions/diverticular-disease/support
5. **The Best Online Therapy for Anxiety of 2024, Tried and tested** https://www.verywellmind.com/the-11-best-online-therapy-companies-for-anxiety-tried-and-tested-8424779
6. **988 Suicide & Crisis Lifeline** https://www.samhsa.gov/find-help/988
7. **Resilience possible in the face of chronic illness diagnosis** https://www.northshore.org/healthy-you/resilience-chronic-illness-diagnosis/

8. **Mental Health and Diverticulitis: Strategies for Managing anxiety and depression** https://calmingblends.com/mental-health-and-diverticulitis-strategies-for-managing-anxiety-and-depression/

9. **Diverticulosis/ Diverticulitis - Support Groups** https://www.medindia.net/health/conditions/diverticulosis-and-diverticulitis-support-groups.htm

10. **65 Healing Affirmations For Chronic Illness - PromptsFirst** https://promptsfirst.com/affirmations-for-chronic-illness/

11. **Surviving diverticulitis: How a health scare transformed this CEO's life** https://www.bswhealth.com/blog/surviving-diverticulitis

12. **Lifestyle Changes for Diverticulosis** https://www.gimedhealth.com/blog/524020-lifestyle-changes-for-diverticulosis/

13. **Managing Diverticular Disease** https://www.eatrightpro.org/news-center/practice-trends/diverticular-disease

14. **Emotional dimensions of chronic disease - PMC** https://pmc.ncbi.nlm.nih.gov/articles/PMC1070773/

15. **AGA Clinical Practice Update on Medical Management of ...** https://www.gastrojournal.org/article/S0016-5085(20)35512-8/fulltext

16. **Diverticulosis & Diverticulitis | ACG** https://gi.org/topics/diverticulosis-and-diverticulitis/

17. **The 9 Best Books on Gut Health** https://www.usenourish.com/blog/gut-health-books

18. **The Sensitive Gut - Harvard Online Courses** https://pll.harvard.edu/course/sensitive-gut

GLOSSARY

Anal: a canal you cannot see

Artery: the study of paintings

Bacteria: back door to cafeteria

Barium: what doctors do when patients die

Benign: what you be after you be eight

Caecum: what happens when you hide'em

Caesarean section: a neighborhood in Rome

CAT scan: searching for kitty

Cauterize: make eye contact with her

Colic: a sheep dog

Coma: a punctuation mark

D&C: where Washington is

Dilate: to live long

Enema: not a friend

Fester: quicker than someone else

Fibula: a small lie

Genital: non-Jewish person

G.I. series: World Series of military baseball

Gullet: What a seabird consumed

Hangnail: what you hang your coat on

Impotent: distinguished, well known

Labor pain: getting hurt at work

Medical staff: a doctor's cane

Morbid: a higher offer than I bid

Nitrates: cheaper than day rates

Node: I knew it

Outpatient: a person who has fainted

Pap smear: a fatherhood test

Pelvis: second cousin to Elvis

Poop: a messy boat deck

Post operative: a letter carrier

Recovery room: place to do upholstery

Rectum: damn near killed him

Secretion: hiding something

Seizure: Roman emperor

Tablet: a small table

Terminal illness: getting sick at the airport

Tumour: one more than one more

Urine: opposite of you're out

Varicose: near by

REFERENCES

Your digestive system and how it works - NIDDK
https://www.niddk.nih.gov/health-information/digestive-diseases/digestive-system-how-it-works

Cohen JS, Sackier JM. Management of colorectal foreign bodies: a retrospective review and report of forty-nine cases. J R Coll Surg Edinb. 1996;41:312-315.

Diverticulosis: what it is, symptoms, causes & treatment
https://my.clevelandclinic.org/health/diseases/24883-diverticulosis

Ravo B, Ger R, Mishrik A, Sackier JM. The treatment of perforated diverticulitis by one stage intracolonic bypass procedure. Surgery. 1987;102(5):771-776.

Abdominal tenderness: causes, symptoms, and treatment
https://www.medicalnewstoday.com/articles/325126

Abdominal quadrants & organs: 4 quadrants, 9 regions
https://simplenursing.com/abdominal-quadrants-organs-four-quadrants-nine-regions/

Diverticulosis vs. diverticulitis: what's the difference?
https://www.templehealth.org/about/blog/diverticulosis-vs-diverticulitis-what-is-the-difference

Diverticulosis. StatPearls
https://www.ncbi.nlm.nih.gov/books/NBK430771/

Pathophysiology and epidemiology of diverticular disease
https://www.ncbi.nlm.nih.gov/pmc/articles/PMC7904337/

Diverticulitis: symptoms and causes
https://www.mayoclinic.org/diseases-conditions/diverticulitis/symptoms-causes/syc-20371758

Misdiagnosis of diverticulitis in patients with irritable bowel syndrome. Mayo Clin Proc. 2016;91(12):1694-1700.
https://www.mayoclinicproceedings.org/article/S0025-6196(16)30511-0/fulltext

IBS vs. diverticulitis: symptoms, causes, treatment, and more
https://www.medicalnewstoday.com/articles/ibs-vs-diverticulitis

Diverticular disease: diagnosis and treatment. Am Fam Physician. 2005;72(7):1229-1234.
https://www.aafp.org/pubs/afp/issues/2005/1001/p1229.html

Uncommon diverticular disease
https://www.ncbi.nlm.nih.gov/pmc/articles/PMC6014836/

Inherited genes linked to higher risk for diverticular disease
https://www.news-medical.net/news/20230704/Inherited-genes-linked-to-higher-risk-for-diverticu-lar-disease-of-intestine.aspx

Peery AF, et al. Diet, ageing and genetic factors in the pathogenesis of diverticulosis. Gut. 2009;58(2):222-228.
https://pmc.ncbi.nlm.nih.gov/articles/PMC2686906/

Eating, diet, & nutrition for diverticular disease. NIDDK
https://www.niddk.nih.gov/health-information/digestive-diseases/diverticulosis-diverticulitis/eating-diet-nutrition

Smoking and alcohol consumption and risk of incident diverticulitis. Clin Gastroenterol Hepatol. 2023;21(11):2520-2529.
https://www.cghjournal.org/article/S1542-3565(23)01001-7/fulltext

Why healthcare advocacy is important
https://publichealth.tulane.edu/blog/healthcare-advocacy/

Communicating with your doctor
https://www.caregiver.org/resource/communicating-your-doctor

Essential questions to ask your doctor | next appointment
https://www.nationaljewish.org/patients-visitors/patient-info/prepare-for-your-appointment/questions-to-ask-your-doctor

Tracking your digestive health with a bullet style journal
https://badgut.org/information-centre/a-z-digestive-topics/bullet-journal/

Diagnosis of diverticular disease. NIDDK
https://www.niddk.nih.gov/health-information/digestive-diseases/diverticulosis-diverticulitis/diagnosis

Is colonoscopy necessary after computed tomography diagnosis of diverticulitis? World J Gastroenterol. 2014;20(41):15139-15145.
https://pmc.ncbi.nlm.nih.gov/articles/PMC4204723/

Sackier JM. Perforated diverticulitis. In: Dudley H, Carter D, Todd IP, Fielding LP, editors. Operative Surgery. London: Butterworth; 1993. Also selected for publication in: Carter DC, Russell RCG, Pitt HA, editors. Rob & Smith's Atlas of General Surgery. London: Chapman & Hall; 1995.

Block GE, Moossa AR, Sackier JM. Principles of resection and anastomosis. In: Block GE, Moossa AR, editors. Operative Colorectal Surgery. Philadelphia: W.B. Saunders; 1994.

Sackier JM. Robotically assisted surgery. In: Steichen FM, Welter R, editors. Minimally Invasive Surgery. 2nd ed. St. Louis: Quality Medical Publishing; 1994.

Sackier JM. Laparoscopic surgery in colorectal disease. In: Corman MR, editor. Colon and Rectal Surgery. Philadelphia: Lippincott; 1998.

Mayo Clinic Minute: tips to make colonoscopy bowel prep easier https://newsnetwork.mayoclinic.org/discussion/mayo-clinic-minute-tips-to-make-colonoscopy-bowel-prep-easier

Understanding your colonoscopy results
https://share.upmc.com/2024/02/understanding-colonoscopy-results/

Diverticular disease: greatest myths and facts https://health.clevelandclinic.org/diverticular-disease-greatest-myths-and-facts

Diverticulosis and diverticulitis
https://www.mayoclinic.org/diseases-conditions/diverticulitis/multimedia/diverticulosis-and-diverticulitis/img-20006098

Long-term risk of acute diverticulitis among patients with diverticulosis. Clin Gastroenterol Hepatol. 2018;16(9):1474-1482.
https://www.ncbi.nlm.nih.gov/pmc/articles/PMC5731451/

Diverticulitis diet: foods to eat, avoid, and more
https://www.healthline.com/health/diverticulitis-diet-list-of-foods-to-avoid

Diverticulitis and stress
https://evinature.com/blog/gut-health/diverticulitis-and-stress-can-stress-trigger-diverticulitis

How to keep a food journal: instructions and tips
https://www.healthline.com/nutrition/food-journaling-instructions-and-tips

Simple lifestyle changes for better gut health
https://integrishealth.org/resources/on-your-health/2023/october/simple-lifestyle-changes-for-better-gut-health

Soluble vs. insoluble fiber: what's the difference?
https://www.healthline.com/health/soluble-vs-insoluble-fiber

High fiber diet for diverticulosis
https://stanfordhealthcare.org/content/dam/SHC/for-patients-component/programs-services/clinical-nutrition-services/docs/pdf-highfiberdietfordiverticulosis.pdf

Dietary fiber: essential for a healthy diet
https://www.mayoclinic.org/healthy-lifestyle/nutrition-and-healthy-eating/in-depth/fiber/art-20043983

Can you take MiraLAX every day?
https://www.singlecare.com/blog/can-you-take-miralax-every-day/

Diverticular disease. Johns Hopkins Medicine
https://www.hopkinsmedicine.org/health/conditions-and-diseases/diverticular-disease

Bowel retraining. MedlinePlus
https://medlineplus.gov/ency/article/003971.htm

Knowles CH, Scott SM, Lunniss PJ. Slow transit constipation: a review of a colonic functional disorder. Neurogastroenterol Motil. 1999;11(3):201-207.
https://www.ncbi.nlm.nih.gov/pmc/articles/PMC2780201/

High and low FODMAP foods
https://www.monashfodmap.com/about-fodmap-and-ibs/high-and-low-fodmap-foods/

Starting the low-FODMAP diet
https://www.verywellhealth.com/how-to-follow-the-low-fodmap-diet-1944680

Koide A, Yamaguchi T, Odaka T, et al. Role of intestinal gas in functional abdominal bloating and distension: a mechanistic review. J Gastroenterol. 2010;45(4):344-352.
https://pmc.ncbi.nlm.nih.gov/articles/PMC3042213/

Setting up a digestive-friendly kitchen in your new home
https://tristategastro.net/setting-up-a-digestive-friendly-kitchen-in-your-new-home

Easy low FODMAP recipes for IBS
https://www.healthline.com/health/22-ibs-friendly-recipes

Alternative products for food intolerances (with recipes!)
https://integrishealth.org/resources/on-your-health/2019/august/alternative-products-for-food-intolerances

Mindful eating. Harvard Health
https://www.health.harvard.edu/staying-healthy/mindful-eating

Home remedies to relieve diverticulitis pain fast
https://www.verywellhealth.com/home-remedies-for-diverticulitis-5268139

Low-residue diet: foods, menus, and more
https://www.webmd.com/ibd-crohns-disease/crohns-disease/low-residue-diet-foods

Diverticulitis diet
https://www.mayoclinic.org/healthy-lifestyle/nutrition-and-healthy-eating/in-depth/diverticulitis-diet/art-20048499

Diverticulitis: diagnosis and treatment
https://www.mayoclinic.org/diseases-conditions/diverticulitis/diagnosis-treatment/drc-20371764

Diverticulitis medication: antibiotics
https://emedicine.medscape.com/article/173388-medication

The best herbs to promote gut health
https://muih.edu/what-is-so-amazing-about-using-herbs-to-promote-gut-health/

Tartaglia D, et al. Minimally invasive management of diverticular disease: a review. World J Gastrointest Surg. 2021;13(2):119-134.
https://pmc.ncbi.nlm.nih.gov/articles/PMC7904339/

Colostomy care. StatPearls
https://www.ncbi.nlm.nih.gov/books/NBK560503/

Ileocecal valve massage for constipation, diverticulitis
https://m.youtube.com/watch?v=e4skK4ygK0w

Benefits of guided imagery for pain management. Beaumont Health
https://www.beaumont.org/services/pain-management-services/benefits-of-guided-imagery-for-pain-management

The health benefits of tai chi. Harvard Health
https://www.health.harvard.edu/staying-healthy/the-health-benefits-of-tai-chi

Zeidan F, et al. Mindfulness meditation–based pain relief: a mechanistic account. J Neurosci. 2016;36(18): 4485–4495.
https://www.ncbi.nlm.nih.gov/pmc/articles/PMC4941786/

Water: how much should you drink every day? Mayo Clinic
https://www.mayoclinic.org/healthy-lifestyle/nutrition-and-healthy-eating/in-depth/water/art-20044256

Hydration and digestion: the link between water and gut health
https://bgapc.com/hydration-and-digestion-gut-health/

The 9 best teas for digestion
https://www.healthline.com/nutrition/tea-for-digestion

The 9 best hydration apps for 2024
https://www.healthline.com/health/hydration-top-iphone-android-apps-drinking-water

How to improve and reset gut health
https://www.healthline.com/health/gut-health

Digestive wellness: the importance of regular check-ups
https://www.biocam.ai/post/digestive-wellness-the-importance-of-regular-check-ups

Fermented foods can add depth to your diet. Harvard Health
https://www.health.harvard.edu/staying-healthy/fermented-foods-can-add-depth-to-your-diet

Mindful eating: nurturing digestive wellness
https://tristategastro.net/mindful-eating-nurturing-digestive-wellness-through-mind-body-connection/

The importance of exercise for digestive health
https://www.gastroconsa.com/the-importance-of-exercise-for-digestive-health/

Five benefits of walking after eating. Doctors Hospital
https://doctors-hospital.net/blog/entry/5-benefits-of-walking-after-eating

Can yoga help aid digestion? 9 poses to try
https://www.healthline.com/nutrition/yoga-posture-for-digestion

Breathing exercises to improve your digestive health. Loyola Medicine
https://www.loyolamedicine.org/newsroom/blog-articles/how-breathing-exercises-relieve-stress-and-improve-digestive-health

Healing gut health: 10 sustainable habits
https://rightnutritionworks.com/gut-health/healing-gut-health-habits/

The SMART way to approach your health goals. Monday Campaigns
https://www.mondaycampaigns.org/healthy-monday/the-smart-way-to-approach-your-health-goals

Foods for diverticulosis and diverticulitis. Johns Hopkins Medicine
https://www.hopkinsmedicine.org/health/wellness-and-prevention/foods-for-diverticulosis-and-diverticulitis

How seasonal changes affect your gut
https://continentalhospitals.com/blog/how-seasonal-changes-affect-your-gut/

How probiotics and prebiotics affect gut health
https://www.healthpartners.com/blog/prebiotic-and-probiotic/

Integrated traditional herbal medicine in the treatment of diverticular disease. Front Pharmacol. 2023;14:10591345.
https://pmc.ncbi.nlm.nih.gov/articles/PMC10591345/

Supplements and your gut health. Mayo Clinic Health System
https://www.mayoclinichealthsystem.org/hometown-health/speaking-of-health/do-supplements-help-or-hurt-gut-health

Kuroki T, et al. A double-blind, randomized, placebo-controlled pilot study of probiotics in diverticular disease. J Clin Biochem Nutr. 2018;63(1):60-65.
https://pmc.ncbi.nlm.nih.gov/articles/PMC6083746/

Hunter JG, Sackier JM. Minimally invasive surgery. New York: McGraw-Hill; 1993.

Arregui M, Sackier JM. Minimal access coloproctology. Oxford: Radcliffe Medical Press; 1995.

Gut health: how deep meditation can improve it. Healthline
https://www.healthline.com/health-news/gut-health-how-deep-meditation-can-improve-it

Meditation and its impact on gut health. Gutbliss
https://gutbliss.com/meditation-its-impact-on-gut-health/

Foster JA, et al. Mindfulness, gut–brain axis, and health-related quality of life. Front Psychiatry. 2024;15:11202893.
https://www.ncbi.nlm.nih.gov/pmc/articles/PMC11202893/

Meditation for beginners. Headspace
https://www.headspace.com/meditation/meditation-for-beginners

Neuroanatomy, parasympathetic nervous system. StatPearls
https://www.ncbi.nlm.nih.gov/books/NBK553141/

Zhu Y, et al. Intervention study of tai chi training on the intestinal flora of middle-aged and elderly women. Front Microbiol. 2023;14:10489434.
https://pmc.ncbi.nlm.nih.gov/articles/PMC10489434/

Two simple Qi Gong postures to boost your internal energy. Holden Qi Gong
https://www.holdenqigong.com/blog/two-simple-qi-gong-postures-to-boost-your-internal-energy

Travelling with diverticular disease/diverticulosis
https://tummytrouble.health.blog/2019/08/07/travelling-with-diverticular-disease-diverticulosis/

The dos and don'ts of managing diverticular disease. Harvard Health
https://www.health.harvard.edu/diseases-and-conditions/the-dos-and-donts-of-managing-diverticular-disease

Fifteen healthy snacks for gut health, according to a dietitian
https://www.health.com/healthy-snack-for-gut-health-7558359

Communicating health needs to employers/teachers. Autism Stay Safe
https://autismstaysafe.org/navigating-healthcare-conversations/communicating-health-needs-to-employers-teachers

Effective patient–physician communication. Obstet Gynecol. 2014;123(2 Pt 1):389-393.
https://www.acog.org/clinical/clinical-guidance/committee-opinion/articles/2014/02/effective-patient-physician-communication

van de Wall BJM, et al. The role of primary care physicians in early diagnosis and treatment of diverticulitis. Ann Gastroenterol. 2014;27(2):147-151.
https://www.ncbi.nlm.nih.gov/pmc/articles/PMC3958525/

Sackier JM. Laparoscopy: applications to colorectal surgery. Semin Colon Rectal Surg. 1992;3(1):2-8.

Colorectal cancer: what you should know about screening. FDA
https://www.fda.gov/consumers/consumer-updates/colorectal-cancer-what-you-should-know-about-screening

Dr Handford's travel tips: diverticular disease & diverticulosis
https://www.goodtogoinsurance.com/medical-travel-insurance/diverticular-disease-diverticulosis

Sackier JM, Slutzki S, Wood CB, Negri M, Moor EV, Halevy A. Laparoscopic endocorporeal mobilization followed by extracorporeal sutureless anastomosis for carcinoma of the left colon. Dis Colon Rectum. 1993;36:610-612.

Effects of aging on the digestive system. Merck Manual
https://www.merckmanuals.com/home/digestive-disorders/biology-of-the-digestive-system/effects-of-aging-on-the-digestive-system

Grossman P, et al. Mindfulness-based stress reduction for people with chronic illness. J Psychosom Res. 2010;68(6): 587–596.
https://pubmed.ncbi.nlm.nih.gov/20815988/

Lifestyle changes for diverticular disease. NYU Langone Health
https://nyulangone.org/conditions/diverticular-disease/treatments/lifestyle-changes-for-diverticular-disease

Peery AF, et al. Emerging evidence and recent controversies in diverticulitis. Curr Opin Gastroenterol. 2022;38(1):50-56.
https://pmc.ncbi.nlm.nih.gov/articles/PMC8713340/

Sackier JM, Wang Y. Robotically assisted laparoscopic surgery: from concept to development. Surg Endosc. 1994;8:63-66.

Made in United States
Troutdale, OR
06/03/2026

49677172R00100